THE 21-DAY SHAPE-UP PROGRAM

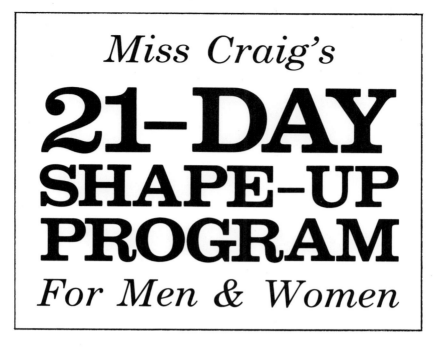

Miss Craig's

21-DAY SHAPE-UP PROGRAM

For Men & Women

A Plan of Natural Movement Exercises for Anyone in Search of a Trim and Healthy Body

by Marjorie Craig

All exercises demonstrated by the author.
Photographs by Frank Foster

Random House/New York

CONTENTS

INTRODUCTION

For the past thirty-three years it has been my pleasure, as well as my profession, to try to find exercise answers for muscular problems as varied in nature as my students have been in age, size and shape. My work began at the Neurological Institute of the Columbia Presbyterian Medical Center, where for seven years my chief concern was aiding men, women and children to rehabilitate muscles which they had damaged in accidents, or lost temporary use of through illness or surgery. My training and experience in teaching people how to reeducate hurt muscles stood me in good stead when I began muscular reeducation of a different sort on my job at Richard Hudnut's, and for the past sixteen years as the supervisor of the Body Department and teacher of private exercise lessons at Elizabeth Arden's in New York.

Literally thousands of very different types of women come to me each year at the Arden Salon, yet they all have one interest in common: *their shape.* Some come to learn exercises which will help them change the shape of their shapes—believing that through exercise they can remold their bodies and rid them of lumps and bumps as they tighten flabby drooping muscles. Others come because they are feeling tense and/or tired and hope that by doing my exercise program they will feel physically fit. Still others come who are in beautiful shape—in form as well as in health—but who are determined through exercising daily to keep themselves that way.

As a teacher who must face her pupils each day rather than one who can be made to vanish at the flick of a TV switch, I have had to think long and hard about my exercise program and be certain that it gets the results I promise. As a consequence, over the years I have invented, adapted, tested, changed and retested hundreds of exercises to meet the needs of *all* my pupils before finally arriving at the complete program which is printed in its entirety for the first time in this book. I did not develop this program for the sake of change or for the sake of being different—though my exercises are different from the gymnastics generally associated with physical-fitness programs and those I was trained to teach as I earned my B. S. in Physical Education at Arnold College (now Bridgeport University). My program became different when I learned through day-to-day experience that gymnastic-type exercises were wrong for most of the people whom I later taught. Fortunately, I quickly saw—as have my clients in the intervening years—that it is not necessary to do the violent exercises which cause one to grunt and groan and in extreme cases to strain muscles, and/or overdevelop them so that bodies become a series of muscular bulges.

There is no stiff-legged or push-up type of calisthenics in my program—which I believe explains why my pupils do not get bad backs or pull ligaments as a penalty for doing exercises to keep in shape. The great majority of the exercises in my program are done while lying on the floor. In this way the maximum results can be obtained with no strain and tension on muscles or on the organs of the body. And the exerciser is not struggling against the pull of gravity. In a sense, gravity will be helping him to get the maximum results with the minimum amount of strain and torture on his part. One of the first things I tell my lady clients is, "Do not do the exercises your husband does; they are too strenuous. Instead let him do yours. If he does, he'll probably feel better and still get the results he wants—a slim, trim figure." My clients have passed my advice along to their husbands—and though men cannot take exercise lessons at Elizabeth Arden's, they can and have learned my program through their wives, or I have personally taught them on weekends at their homes.

Because I give only private instructions, the number of half-hour exercise lessons I can give each day is necessarily limited. At my clients' urging I am therefore now making my program available to the public. I hope everyone will find it as useful as my loyal, conscientious pupils have.

As the teacher, I have posed to illustrate the movements for all the exercises in this book, but this does not mean they are exclusively for women. All the exercises included in the 21-Day Shape-Up Program, and those in the other sections that answer special needs, will be beneficial to men as well as to women— and even for children.

I feel that the readers of this book, be they male or female, should understand the reasons they should exercise and what results they might expect if they follow my program, so I have culled questions most frequently asked by my clients and present them here along with the answers I give.

Why Exercise?
The shape of your body depends first upon your bone structure— your skeleton. One's skeletal structure is clothed with fat and muscle, and it is this clothing which accounts for most of the body's weight. But whether or not one is overweight, it is the condition of the body's muscles that finally determines whether one has a smooth contour or one with bulges or sagging flesh.

More than one half of the human body is comprised of muscle. Every muscle is there to be used. Muscles work together in pairs and in groups. When one group of muscles contracts, the opposite group relaxes. No single muscle works alone. If groups of muscles are not used, or used too little, they tend to deteriorate and lose their tone—that is, strength, firmness and elasticity. Muscles which are not used enough become weak and flabby, and sag. If there is extra fat in the body, it will gravitate to, and settle around, muscles which are not in tone. Weak and flabby muscles cannot break up fat and move it out of the system. When fat settles around muscles, they stretch, and stretched muscles sag, causing surrounding tissues to sag. The fat may make the body look firm, but a weight loss will prove that it isn't. Weight loss cannot bring sagging muscles back into tone— only exercise can. The *right* exercises. For muscles can be over-developed as well as underdeveloped. If muscles are constantly tensed, or forced to carry workloads meant for larger muscles, muscles will become bigger. The body does not need big, over-developed muscles to function well. As a matter of fact, when muscles become too big they get in the way of other muscles and slow down movements, and in addition, cause body bulges.

Muscles produce all body movements, maintain body positions (standing, sitting, bending, etc.), form a natural girdle to hold internal organs in their correct positions, push food along the digestive tract, suck air into the lungs and regulate blood pressure. The heart itself is a muscular pump. There are more than 600 muscles in the body. They all need to be exercised (used) regularly and properly to keep them healthy. This is why one needs to purposefully exercise muscles in all parts of the body every single day. They should be exercised without tenseness and strain (so they do not become overdeveloped). They should be contracted and extended easily and smoothly only as far as they can comfortably go. Only in this way can firmness and tone be developed in the entire length of the muscles without creating body bulges. "There is strong authoritative support," says the President's Council on Physical Fitness, "for the concept that regular exercise can help prevent degenerative diseases and slow down the physical deterioration that accompanies aging." Therefore, it would seem apparent from a health point of view that it is as important to keep your muscles in tone as it is to brush your teeth, comb your hair or eat. Certainly, from the point of view of physical appearance, my many clients have proved again and again that one can sculpture his body to his liking— the only limitation being the bone structure—by doing my recommended program daily. Exercise—the right kind, that is—is a must for anyone who wants to look well and feel well.

How Much Time Is Required for Exercises?
Though some exercise programs purport that one can condition the body in just ten minutes a day, I have never found this to be the case. There is no way yet discovered, be it jogging, walking, isometrics, gymnastics, sports—such as swimming, tennis, golf—or a machine that exercises for you, which will condition and contour the total body in ten minutes a day. To get in condition and stay in condition, one must systematically exercise muscles in all parts of the body in order to correct faulty posture, to reduce certain areas and to firm flabby muscles in other areas, and this is what my program insures. There is no use kidding yourself or hoping for miracles; conditioning, and keeping in condition, requires time.

I have found that at least thirty minutes of exercise every day are required to condition the body, correct posture and bring the whole body into contour. Once the body is conditioned and perfectly contoured, a half hour of exercise every day is still necessary to keep it that way, and my program is geared for this amount of time. Exercise should be part of everyone's daily routine. And I know that those who do my program conscientiously always feel so much better and always look so much better that they *always* think it is time well spent. And the "time" cloud has another silver lining—the mere minutes you spend exercising each day may well add "time" to your life.

How Long Does It Take to Get in Shape?

If you do my exercise program conscientiously daily, you will see results in a week's time (provided you do not increase your food intake just because you are exercising), and will probably feel better after your very first exercise session. I have clients who without dieting have lost an inch in measurements in various parts of their body after doing the total program for two weeks. Clients who have combined my program with a reasonable diet have lost as much as an inch in various parts of their body in one week's time. Every individual responds differently, according to the physiology of the body. The amount of time it will take you to bring your total body into perfect contour, to firm the muscles and increase their strength and flexibility depends, of course, upon the shape you are in when you start the program. If you are like so many people who have said to me, "I have exercised all my life but nothing happened," then you probably have been doing the wrong type of exercises. I will tell you what I have told the others, and that is, "If you do these exercises and stick to them, you can get the results you desire." Any figure problem (except those caused by a physical deformity) can be corrected if you do the right exercises.

What About "Spot" Exercising?

It is true that special-area exercises, such as those for hips, thighs, abdomen, etc., bring other muscles into action, but the only way one can be sure one is toning muscles in all parts of the body is by following a systematic program. I always tell my clients (as I have the readers of this book) which parts of the body a given exercise is directed to, but this does not—and should not—imply that I believe area exercises should be done to the exclusion of the total program I recommend. By describing what portions of the body each exercise is intended to help, I hope to permit my unseen clients to decide intelligently whether to decrease the number of times they do certain exercises. For example, if some necessary movements of your daily routine have kept certain portions of your body—say, your hips—in good shape, you can decrease—note, I did not say eliminate—the number of times you do the exercises intended to tone the muscles in the hip area, and use these gained minutes to add exercises from the "Five for Good Measure" section for those portions of your body which may not be as well toned by some one of your daily activities.

Can Weight Be Lost by Exercising?

According to studies made by Dr. Jean Mayer, senior member of the faculty of the Department of Nutrition of the Harvard School of Public Health, "regular and moderate exercise exerts a beneficial effect on body weight . . . one half hour of exercise each day can keep off or take off as much as twenty-six pounds a year." My own experience has proven that exercise breaks up fat around lazy muscles. If you need to lose a lot of weight, as well as measurements, exercise alone will not necessarily make your weight decrease, though in time the extra weight you carry will be reproportioned as muscles tighten and firm, and thus bulges of fat will disappear and your contour will be smoother. Just by correcting bad posture you can give the appearance of being ten pounds thinner than you really are.

If your body has a great deal of flabby fat on it, you may be cheered to know that with exercise soft fat will break up more quickly than solid, hard fat. Those who have solid fat on their bodies will need to break up the fat deposits with diet and exercise. As they lose weight and their measurements decrease, they will notice that as the fat breaks up, it gradually softens before it goes away. Just keep exercising and your body will eventually firm and tighten.

THE 21-DAY SHAPE-UP PROGRAM

SECTION I

THE 21-DAY SHAPE-UP PROGRAM

The charts at the bottom of Exercises 1 through 35 are to guide you day by day through the 21-Day Shape-Up Program and on to the Maintenance level.

The charts reflect the changes and additions to be made in the program day by day.

The day you are to start a new exercise is delineated with a spotlighted number.

	1st Day	2nd Day	3rd Day	20th Day	21st Day	Maintenance
Number of times	6	6	6	10	10	10

The numerals in this row indicate the number of times each exercise is to be done daily.

Start your program each day with Exercise 1 and work on through until you've completed the day's program. Once an exercise has been introduced, it will become part of all of the subsequent days' programs. On some days new exercises will be added, on others only the number of times you do certain exercises will vary. So that there can be no question as to which day of the program you are working on, record your progress by crossing off the day on the charts as you complete each exercise.

When you reach the Maintenance level on the chart, it will take you about 30 minutes a day to work through the program. You cannot be sure of exercising muscles in all parts of the body unless you do all of the exercises in the 21-Day Shape-Up Program.

Of course, every person should check with his personal physician before beginning any exercise program. If you are not used to exercising at all, get his advice as to your individual ability to move through the program. Some of my clients have learned all 35 exercises in the 21-Day Shape-Up Program in a week's time. Depending upon your physical condition and whether you are used to exercising, you, too, can move along at an even more rapid rate than is suggested by the charts. If you do the exercises slowly and with relaxed motions, as suggested, you will not get sore muscles and become stiff even if you learn and do all 35 exercises the first week. The quicker you learn the total program, the quicker you will see results.

But when exercising, never force any movement so that a muscle feels strained and never hurry through your exercises. If time is a factor, do half the program in the morning and the rest when you have more time. The exercises do not have to be done in the order they are presented here, but I think it is a good order, because you can move from lying on the floor to a sitting position and on to standing position to finish off, and it is arranged to give muscles rest periods as you move from exercise to exercise. If a muscle feels tired before you have done the recommended number of times of any exercise, rest a few seconds, then complete it.

Measurements

Before you start your 21-Day Shape-Up Program, take your measurements. Measure the portions of your body as indicated on the facing page. (Always measure the same limb, for right and left limb measurements may be different.) Record the measurements of chest, upper arm, bust, waist, abdomen, upper hips, lower hips, top thigh, mid-thigh, knee, calf and ankle, along with the date you took the measurements. Measure again 10 days after starting the program and every 10 days thereafter until you reach perfect proportions. These measurements will guide you to which exercises in the "Five for Good Measure" section you may need to supplement your exercise program. As your measurements change, your program of supplementary exercises may need to be changed. Once you've reached perfect proportions, check your measurements once a month.

PERFECT PROPORTIONS

For Women:

Bust measurement and lower hip measurement should be the same; the waist 10 inches less than lower hips and the bust.

For Men:

Chest measurement should be somewhat larger, and waist should be somewhat smaller, than lower hips.

WHERE TO MEASURE:

CHEST - under armpits, straight around

UPPER ARM - 4" down from armpit, then around

BUST - straight across back and over the fullest part of bust

WAIST - smallest part

ABDOMEN - across the navel, around back, below waist

UPPER HIPS - halfway between abdomen and lower hip

LOWER HIPS - around the largest part of buttocks

TOP THIGH - up under leg as high as possible, and straight around

MID-THIGH - halfway between top-thigh measure and knee

KNEE - around the middle

CALF - around the largest part

ANKLE - around the smallest part, just above ankle bone

Equipment

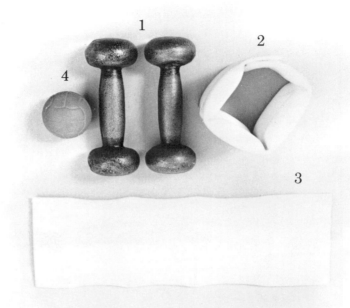

You can proceed with the 21-Day Shape-Up Program without purchasing any special equipment, but for those interested in shaping up more easily and quickly, I would recommend their buying certain items, namely, dumbbells (1), ankle weights (2 & 3), sponge rubber ball (4). For the total list of equipment needed, most of which is readily available at home, see below.

WEIGHTS:

Using weights in conjunction with certain exercises can hasten the strengthening and firming of muscles and bring the body into contour more quickly. Weights should be used only for the exercises which specifically call for them, and no greater poundage of weights than those called for should be used. The exerciser will be using weights held in the hand during the first week of the program. Ankle weights will be called for after the Maintenance level of the 21-Day Shape-Up Program has been reached. They should not be used before this time.

A person who has a history of either lower-back or neck-vertebrae problems should check with his physician before using weights. If for any reason weights are not used in the exercise program, it will be necessary, where weights have been recommended, to double the amount of times the exercises are done.

The weights I suggest are:

Dumbbells: The type of dumbbells I have found to be most practical are those made of cast iron, for they are perfectly balanced and easy to handle (see figure 1). Women should use a pair of dumbbells which weigh 3 pounds each. Men can use a pair of dumbbells which weigh 5 pounds each. It is not necessary to use heavier weights unless the exerciser wants to build bulging muscles. Work with dumbbells only when in a prone position, for using weights while sitting or standing will thicken neck muscles.

Ankle Weights: The type of ankle weights I have found to be the most practical are long leather-like bags filled with sand. These weights have self-adhering ends which means they will hold tightly around various ankle sizes. Ankle weights come in many poundages, but I recommend a pair weighing 3 pounds each (weight strips closed: see figure 2; weight strips open: see figure 3).

The ankle weights and the dumbbells are generally available at sporting-goods stores. Dumbbells sell for about 30¢ a pound. Ankle weights are priced at about $2 a pound.

SPONGE RUBBER BALL:

Using a rubber ball in conjunction with specific exercises will tone certain muscles more quickly because its use necessitates a stronger contraction of these muscles. The ball (see figure 4) should be slightly smaller than a tennis ball (about 2″ in diameter), and one that can be easily held between the heels of the hands. This type of ball is available in most toy and dime stores.

TURKISH TOWELS:

Two bath towels rolled together, to be placed under the buttocks, will be required for certain exercises. Towels rolled together and used in this manner will protect muscles of the lower back from strain while doing exercises for conditioning thigh and leg muscles. Whenever the towels are needed, explicit directions are given—*and they should always be used.*

EXERCISE MAT:

You should not exercise on the floor (even on a rug) without a mat. If you do, you can get black and blue spots and/or irritate the skin with rug burns. It is not necessary to buy a mat; instead use a padded mattress cover, a beach mat or a folded blanket.

EXERCISE SUIT:

You should never exercise in clothing that restricts your movements. If a woman feels it is necessary to wear a brassiere, it should be a loose one. The exercise suits I recommend are leotards with long sleeves for women and children, and loose, non-rubberized sweatsuits for men.

MUSIC:

Exercises should be done smoothly and rhythmically, so it is advisable to play music as you exercise. You can use records, tapes, radio or television as your source of music. I recommend phonograph records or tapes, so that you can select music which is even-tempoed—that is, not too fast, not too slow. An example of this is Frank Sinatra's recording of "Young in Heart."

FULL-LENGTH MIRROR:

If you do exercises in front of a full-length mirror, you will be able to check your movements. Only in this way can you be sure that you are not stiffening arms or legs, hunching shoulders or holding your head at the wrong angle.

SELF-DETERMINATION:

This only YOU can supply. Determine to do—and DO— the exercises every day. With self-determination this program can help you become the shape you want to be. And <u>now</u> is the time to begin.

1 *"Right, Left, and Center"*

FOR THE NECK / PART I

**TO RELIEVE TENSION AND PAIN, PREVENT OR CORRECT
DOUBLE CHIN, IMPROVE JAW OUTLINE AND HEAD CARRIAGE**

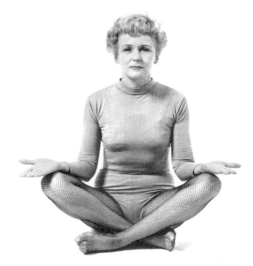

1. Sit on a chair in front of a mirror. Feet flat on floor. Hands on knees. Palms up. Or sit tailor-fashion on floor, as shown. Pull ribs up. Pull abdomen in. Keep spine straight. Pull shoulders back and down. Chin at right angle to neck. Maintain this basic position throughout neck exercises.

2. Keep chin level. *Slowly* turn head toward left shoulder. Remember: *Turn head slowly. Do not jerk head.*

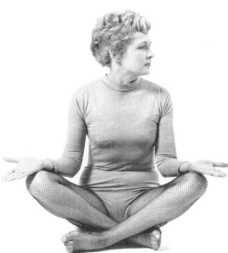

	1st Day	2nd Day	3rd Day	4th Day	5th Day	6th Day	7th Day	8th Day	9th Day	10th Day	11th Day
Number of times	4	4	4	4	6	6	8	8	8	8	6

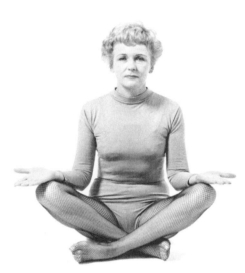

3. Slowly return head to center. Pause. Now give your neck an extra stretch and at the same time pull your shoulders down even more, so that it feels as though someone's hands were pressing down on them. In stretching neck up, remember to keep chin at right angle to body. Hold stretch. Relax.

4. Slowly turn head toward right shoulder. Check in mirror to see you are keeping chin at right angle to body.

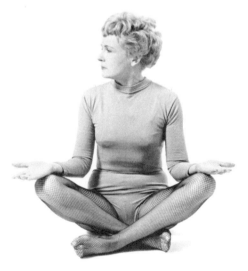

5. Slowly return head to center. Again, stretch neck up and pull shoulders down, as in No. 3.

✓ chart for number of times to do exercise.

2th Day	13th Day	14th Day	15th Day	16th Day	17th Day	18th Day	19th Day	20th Day	21st Day	Maintenance
6	8	8	6	6	6	8	8	8	8	8

"Ear to Shoulder" FOR THE NECK / PART II

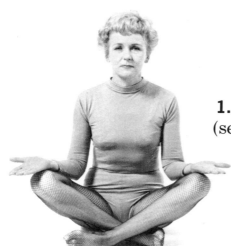

1. Assume basic position (see Part 1).

2. Bend your head to the left. Ear going toward left shoulder. Don't force it. Don't lift shoulder to meet ear.

	1st Day	2nd Day	3rd Day	4th Day	5th Day	6th Day	7th Day	8th Day	9th Day	10th Day	11th Day
Number of times	4	4	4	4	6	6	8	8	8	8	6

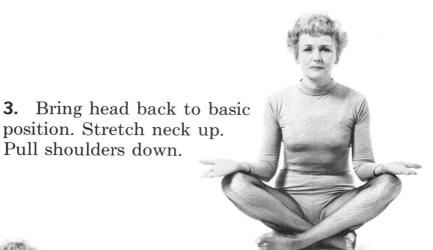

3. Bring head back to basic position. Stretch neck up. Pull shoulders down.

4. Bend your head to the right. Ear going toward right shoulder.

5. Head up. Stretch neck up. Pull shoulders down.

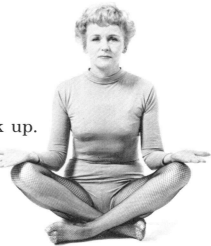

√ chart for number of times to do exercise.

12th Day	13th Day	14th Day	15th Day	16th Day	17th Day	18th Day	19th Day	20th Day	21st Day	Maintenance
6	8	8	6	6	6	8	8	8	8	8

"Head Droop" FOR THE NECK / PART III

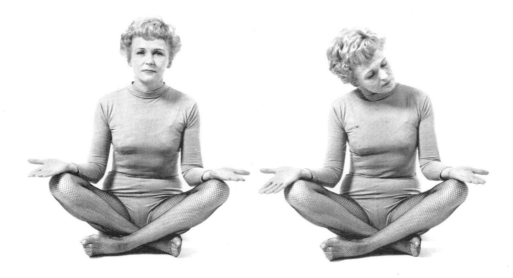

1. Assume basic position.

2. Turn head slightly toward left and let head fall slowly.

3. Bring head back to basic position. Stretch neck up. Pull shoulders down.

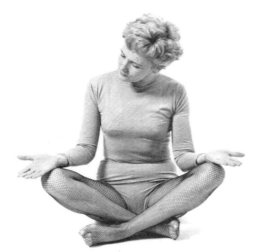

4. Turn head slightly toward right and let head fall slowly.

5. Bring head back up. Stretch neck up. Pull shoulders down.

✓ chart for number of times to do exercise.

	1st Day	2nd Day	3rd Day	4th Day	5th Day	6th Day	7th Day	8th Day	9th Day	10th Day	11th Day
Number of times	4	4	4	4	6	6	8	8	8	8	6

"Head Back" FOR THE NECK / PART IV

1. Assume basic position.

2. Let your head drop back.

3. Slowly lift head as if pulling it up by the top of your ears. Lift ears up away from your shoulders until chin is at right angle to neck. Pull shoulders down.

✓ chart for number of times to do exercise.

"Head Roll" FOR THE NECK / PART V

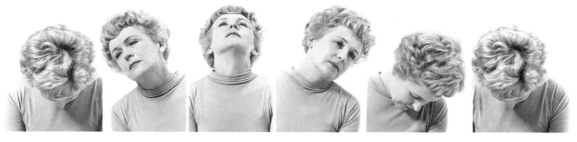

1. Rest chin on chest. 2. Slowly roll head to right shoulder. 3. Roll it to the back. 4. Continue to circle head onto left shoulder. 5. Circle it on to... 6. Starting position. Do entire head roll with a slow, relaxed, continuous motion.

Do exercise 3 times, then reverse circle for 3 times.

12th Day	13th Day	14th Day	15th Day	16th Day	17th Day	18th Day	19th Day	20th Day	21st Day	Maintenance
6	8	8	6	6	6	8	8	8	8	8

2 *"Full Body Stretch"*

TO STRETCH MUSCLES IN WAISTLINE, UPPER HIPS, ABDOMEN AND BACK

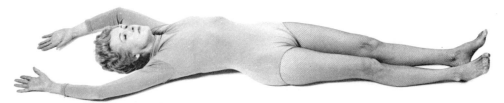

1. Lie down on the floor on your back. Extend both arms along the floor over the head. Turn palms up. Legs straight but relaxed.

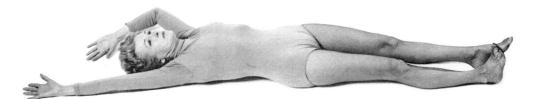

2. Stretch up with your right arm, and at the same time stretch down with *heel* of right leg. (Don't point your toe.) *Stretch.* Pull, pull, pull. Then relax.

	1st Day	2nd Day	3rd Day	4th Day	5th Day	6th Day	7th Day	8th Day	9th Day	10th Day	11th Day
Number of times	6	6	6	8	8	8	10	10	10	10	8

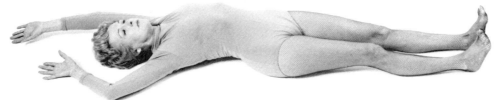

3. Stretch up with left arm and down with left *heel*. *Stretch.* Pull, pull, pull. Then relax.

Checkpoint: During this exercise you should feel your rib cage moving up, and should feel a pull in your upper arm and calf of leg. Remember to keep your neck and elbows relaxed.

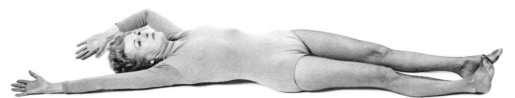

4. Again stretch up with right arm and down with right heel.

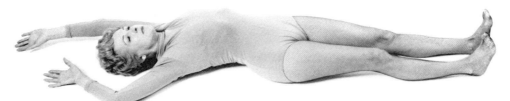

5. Stretch up with left arm, down with left heel.

Repeat these movements, but this time, relaxed and loose.

√ chart for number of times to do exercise.

12th Day	13th Day	14th Day	15th Day	16th Day	17th Day	18th Day	19th Day	20th Day	21st Day	Maintenance
8	8	10	10	8	8	8	10	10	10	10

3 *"Opposite Arm and Leg Touch"*

TO LENGTHEN WAISTLINE, REDUCE UPPER HIPS AND FLATTEN UPPER BACK

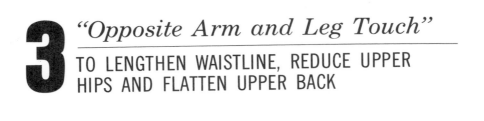

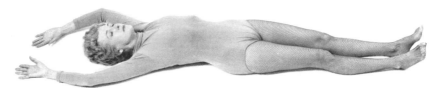

1. Lie on the floor on your back. Extend arms over the head on floor in a relaxed position. Palms turned up. Legs straight but relaxed.

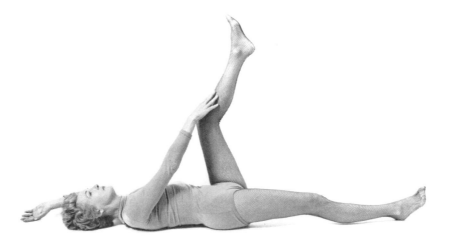

2. Keeping your head and shoulders on floor, raise your right arm and left leg up toward ceiling. Touch right hand to left leg (DO NOT STRAIN to touch toes. Keep knees relaxed), then lower arm, keeping elbow slightly bent, and leg to floor.

	1st Day	2nd Day	3rd Day	4th Day	5th Day	6th Day	7th Day	8th Day	9th Day	10th Day	11th Day
Number of times	10	10	10	10	12	14	18	20	20	20	20

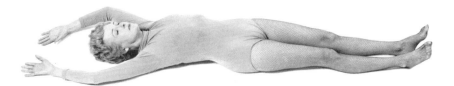

3. With both elbows slightly bent, press arms toward floor. Never force arms back further than they want to go. Try not to arch your back as you press arms down.

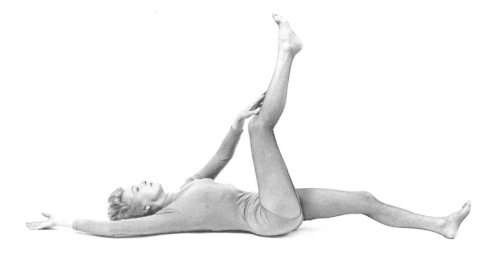

4. Next, raise other arm and leg. Touch, and down. Again press arms toward floor.

√   chart for number of times to do exercise.

2th Day	13th Day	14th Day	15th Day	16th Day	17th Day	18th Day	19th Day	20th Day	21st Day	Maintenance
20	20	20	20	20	18	20	20	20	20	20

4 *"Side Stretch"*

TO REDUCE WAISTLINE, UPPER HIPS AND AROUND ARM SOCKETS

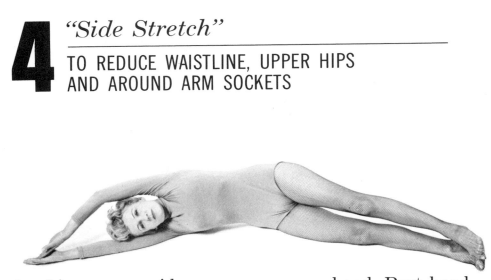

1. Lie on your side, arms over your head. Rest head on underneath arm. *Palms* of *both hands* are turned *up*. Bring both legs forward so you are in a slight semi-circle position. Trunk of body is slightly bent, but legs are kept straight.

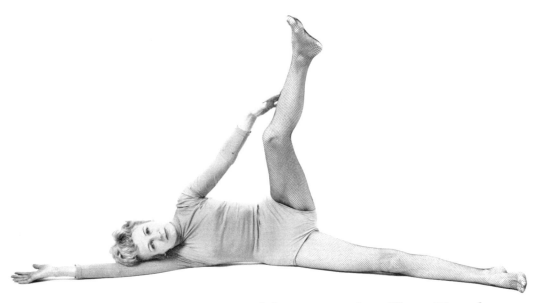

2. Raise your top arm and leg toward ceiling. Touch hand to leg. (Don't try to touch toes.) Return arm and leg to original position. Palms up.

	1st Day	2nd Day	3rd Day	4th Day	5th Day	6th Day	7th Day	8th Day	9th Day	10th Day	11th Day
Number of times	8	8	8	8	10	10	12	15	15	15	15

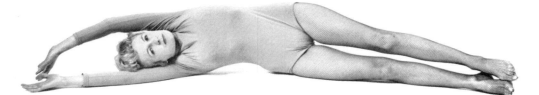

3. When arm and leg return to original position, stretch top arm up behind your head. Stretch as far as you can— pull, pull, pulling your rib cage away from your hips.

√   chart for number of times to do exercise.

After exercising required number of times on one side, turn over and do exercise on other side.

The day will come when during the stretch you will see daylight between your waist and the floor. Then you'll know you are making progress.

2th Day	13th Day	14th Day	15th Day	16th Day	17th Day	18th Day	19th Day	20th Day	21st Day	Maintenance
15	15	12	15	15	12	15	15	15	15	15

5 *"Figure Eight"*

TO REDUCE UPPER HIPS, WAIST AND ABDOMEN

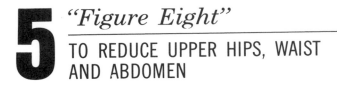

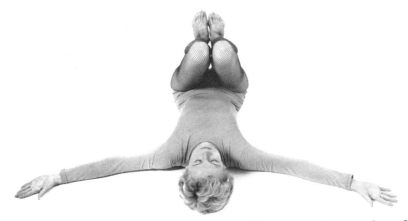

1. Lie on your back, arms extended on floor, shoulder level. Palms turned up. Bend knees up over your chest.

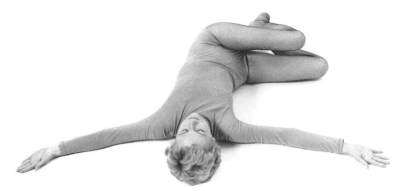

2. Keeping knees together, drop both knees to right side, all the way to the floor, and directly out from hips. Keep arms as close to floor as possible.

	1st Day	2nd Day	3rd Day	4th Day	5th Day	6th Day	7th Day	8th Day	9th Day	10th Day	11 Da
Number of times	10	12	14	16	16	18	20	26	26	26	2

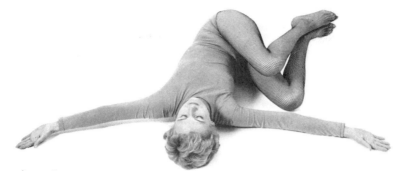

3. Keeping knees on the floor, pull them up toward elbow. Hold. From this pulled-up position:

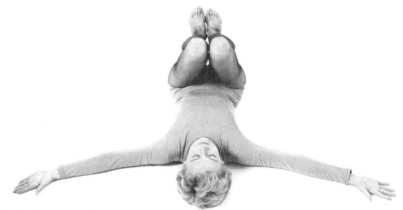

4. Roll knees back over your chest. Hold.

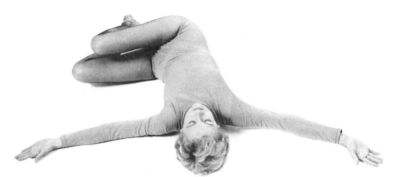

5. Drop both knees to left side directly out from hips; pull knees up toward elbow. Hold. Bring knees back over chest. Hold.

✓ chart for number of times to do exercise.

2th Day	13th Day	14th Day	15th Day	16th Day	17th Day	18th Day	19th Day	20th Day	21st Day	Maintenance
24	24	26	26	24	26	26	24	26	26	26

6 *"Biking Side by Side"*

TO REDUCE FAT ON THIGHS, KNEES, CALVES AND ANKLES

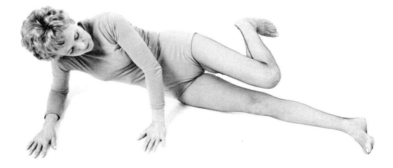

1. Lie down on your side with body in slight semicircle position, with the upper part of body raised and supported on elbow of underneath arm and hand of top arm.

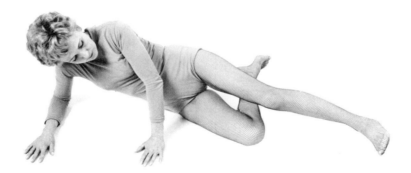

2. With both legs raised about 2″ off floor, bend and straighten legs, first one, then the other, as if you were peddling a bicycle. Pull your toes up and heels

	1st Day	2nd Day	3rd Day	4th Day	5th Day	6th Day	7th Day	8th Day	9th Day	10th Day	11th Day
Number of times	18	20	20	22	25	25	30	30	30	30	30

down and "pump" with your feet in this position. You will then get a pull in the calves of your legs. As you "bicycle," adjust your position on your arms so that you literally massage the side of the upper thigh with each cycling movement.

√   chart for number of times. (Count each time right leg comes up as one complete cycle.) Then roll over and "bicycle" on other side for same number of times.

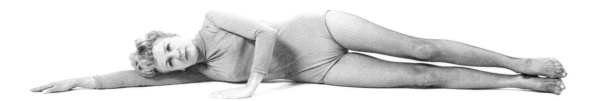

If you do not have a heavy-thigh problem, you will not need to raise the upper portion of body while cycling. Instead, lie on the floor on your side, with head resting on outstretched underneath arm. Place hand of other arm on the floor in front of chest for support. Raise legs 2″ off floor and do exercise.

> NOTE: You will get more benefit from cycling on the floor than from a real bike ride. Real biking can build bulging muscles in the legs. Your simulated ride *tones* muscles and helps reduce upper-thigh bulges.

2th Day	13th Day	14th Day	15th Day	16th Day	17th Day	18th Day	19th Day	20th Day	21st Day	Maintenance
30	30	25	30	30	30	30	30	30	30	30

7 *"Leg Cross-Over"*

TO REDUCE WAIST AND UPPER HIPS

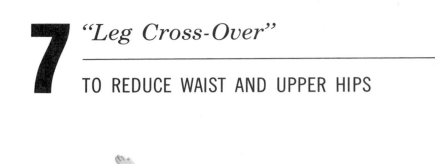

1. Lie on your back, arms extended on floor, shoulder level. Palms turned up. Legs straight and together.

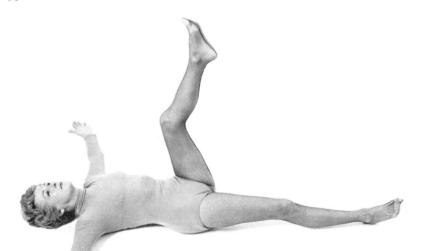

2. Raise left leg up, with knee slightly bent, toward ceiling.

	1st Day	2nd Day	3rd Day	4th Day	5th Day	6th Day	7th Day	8th Day	9th Day	10th Day	11th Day
Number of times	8	8	10	10	10	12	14	18	18	18	20

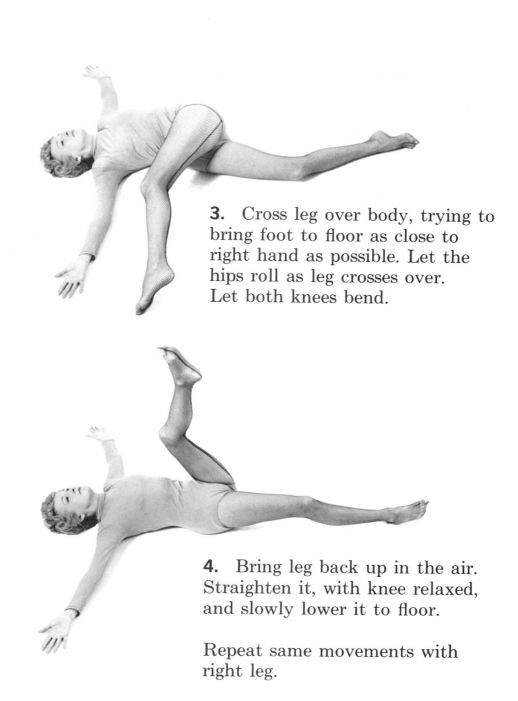

3. Cross leg over body, trying to bring foot to floor as close to right hand as possible. Let the hips roll as leg crosses over. Let both knees bend.

4. Bring leg back up in the air. Straighten it, with knee relaxed, and slowly lower it to floor.

Repeat same movements with right leg.

Throughout this exercise, keep both knees relaxed. Keep shoulders on the floor.

✓ chart for number of times to do exercise with each leg.

2th Day	13th Day	14th Day	15th Day	16th Day	17th Day	18th Day	19th Day	20th Day	21st Day	Maintenance
20	18	20	20	18	18	18	18	20	20	20

8 *"Upper Hip Roll"*

TO REDUCE UPPER HIPS AND WAIST

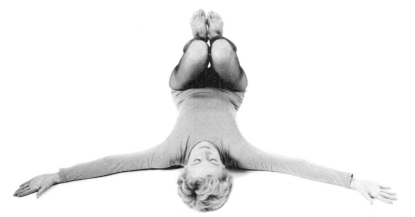

1. Lie on your back, arms extended on floor, shoulder level. Palms turned up. Bend knees up over your chest.

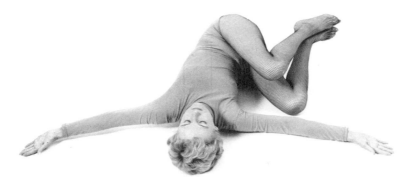

2. Keeping your knees together, roll them over to the floor as close to your right elbow as possible.

	1st Day	2nd Day	3rd Day	4th Day	5th Day	6th Day	7th Day	8th Day	9th Day	10th Day	11th Day
Number of times	8	8	10	10	12	12	14	14	16	18	20

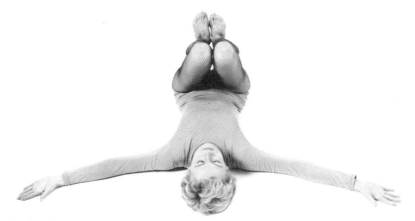

3. Roll knees back to your chest. Hold.

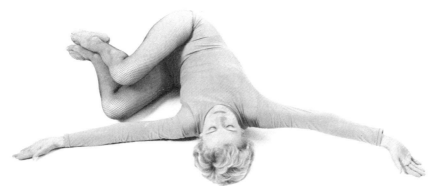

4. Then bring knees over to your left elbow.

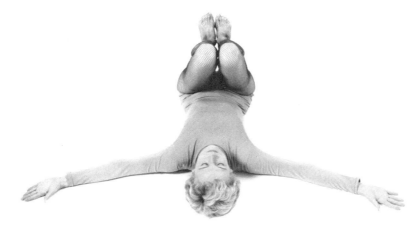

5. Roll knees back to chest. Hold.
✓ chart for number of times to do exercise.

12th Day	13th Day	14th Day	15th Day	16th Day	17th Day	18th Day	19th Day	20th Day	21st Day	Maintenance
20	20	18	20	18	20	18	18	20	20	20

9 "The Basis of Posture"

FOR ALIGNING AND STRAIGHTENING THE SPINE

NOTE: Incorrect posture can be the cause of a protruding abdomen, thick waistline, sagging busts, protruding hips, stooped shoulders, double chin, short neck, knock-knees, bowlegs and flat feet. Incorrect posture is also the cause of many backaches, stiff necks and headaches. To obtain perfect posture while standing and sitting, you're going to start toning your posture muscles while lying on the floor.

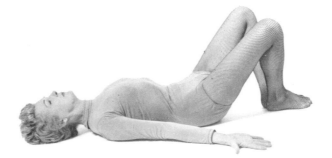

1. Bend your knees. Place feet together on the floor, close to hips. Keep knees slightly apart. Place arms on floor at your sides. Palms turned up.

	1st Day	2nd Day	3rd Day	4th Day	5th Day	6th Day	7th Day	8th Day	9th Day	10th Day	11th Day
Number of times	4	4	4	3	4	4	5	4	4	3	4

2. Waist back. Ribs up. Ears up. Shoulders back and down. Relax.

These are the key phrases which appear in all of the posture exercises. Memorize these phrases and their meanings. Only by acting upon them can you have perfect posture, and thus a perfect figure.

Waist back. This means: With a rolling hip movement, pull your pelvis back so that the small of your back at the waistline touches the floor.

Ribs up. This means: Pull your ribs up away from your hip bones so that you get the greatest distance possible between ribs and hip bones without lifting your spine from the floor.

Ears up. This means: Feel as if someone is holding the top of your ears and is thus stretching your neck up away from your shoulders while you are keeping your chin at a right angle to your neck.

Shoulders back and down. This means: Keep your shoulders as flat on the floor as you can, and at the same time pull them down toward your feet; feel as though your arms were being pulled by your little fingers.

Say and Do the key phrases.

√ chart for number of times.

12th Day	13th Day	14th Day	15th Day	16th Day	17th Day	18th Day	19th Day	20th Day	21st Day	Maintenance
4	4	4	4	4	4	5	5	5	5	5

10 *"Spine Lift"*

TO STRAIGHTEN SPINE AND ELIMINATE "DOWAGER'S HUMP"

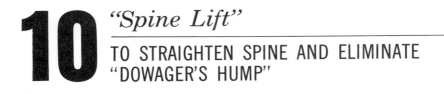

1. Lie on your back, arms at sides. Palms up. Bend your knees and place feet on floor close to hips. Feet together. Knees slightly apart.

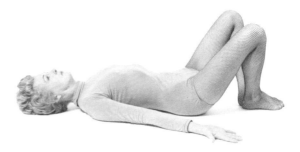

2. Now (as explained in previous exercise):

Waist back.
Ribs up.
Ears up.
Shoulders back and down.

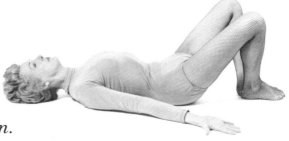

3. Now slowly lift spine off floor, one vertebra at a time, starting with the coccyx (the base of the spine). Up, up, up, until entire body is raised and weight rests on shoulders, neck, head and feet.

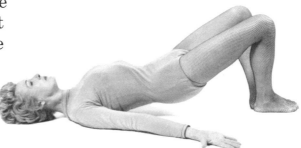

	1st Day	2nd Day	3rd Day	4th Day	5th Day	6th Day	7th Day	8th Day	9th Day	10th Day	11th Day
Number of times	3	3	3	4	4	5	5	5	4	4	5

4. Now press neck back on floor. Don't press chin down. Keep it at right angle to neck. Keep shoulders pulled down.

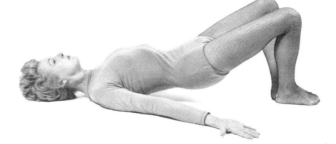

5. Now come down slowly, one vertebra at a time, starting at the top. Drop, drop, drop.

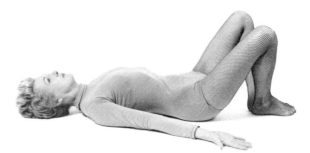

6. Keep hips raised until you lower small of back to floor, then bring hips down.

Relax.

✓ chart for number of times to do exercise.

12th Day	13th Day	14th Day	15th Day	16th Day	17th Day	18th Day	19th Day	20th Day	21st Day	Maintenance
5	4	4	4	4	4	5	5	5	5	5

11 *"Leg Lift"*

TO STRENGTHEN MUSCLES IN PELVIS AND ABDOMEN

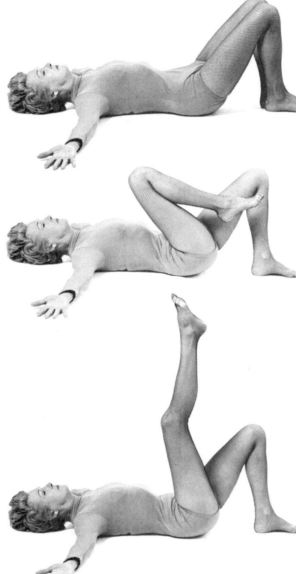

1. Lie on your back, arms extended on floor, shoulder level. Palms up. Bend knees. Place feet on floor close to hips. Feet together. Knees slightly apart.

2. NOW: *Waist back. Ribs up. Ears up. Shoulders back and down.* Holding this position, bend your right knee up toward your chest.

3. Raise the right leg, straightening it as you do so.

	1st Day	2nd Day	3rd Day	4th Day	5th Day	6th Day	7th Day	8th Day	9th Day	10th Day	11th Day
Number of times	4	6	6	6	6	6	4	4	6	6	6

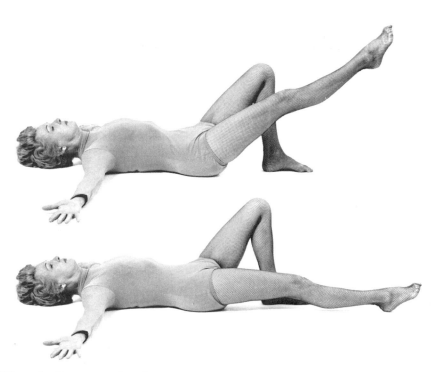

4. *Slowly* lower the leg down to the floor, *keeping spine on the floor* and *stomach pulled in tight.*

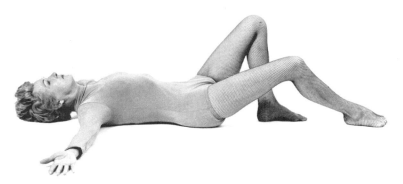

5. Then slowly bend the knee and return leg to its starting position.

Repeat same movements with left leg.

✓ chart for number of times to do exercise.

12th Day	13th Day	14th Day	15th Day	16th Day	17th Day	18th Day	19th Day	20th Day	21st Day	Maintenance
6	4	4	6	6	6	6	4	6	6	6

12

"Inhale—Exhale"

TO FIRM AND FLATTEN ABDOMEN

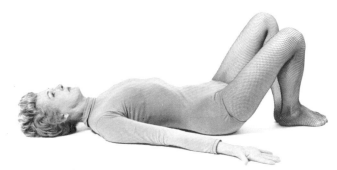

1. Lie on your back, knees bent, feet together on floor close to hips. Keep knees slightly apart. Arms at sides. Palms up.

> Now:
> *Waist back.*
> *Ribs up.*
> *Ears up.*
> *Shoulders back and down.*

	1st Day	2nd Day	3rd Day	4th Day	5th Day	6th Day	7th Day	8th Day	9th Day	10th Day	11th Day
Number of times	4	4	4	4	4	5	4	4	4	5	5

2. Blow all the air you can out of your lungs. Compress your lips and hold your breath.

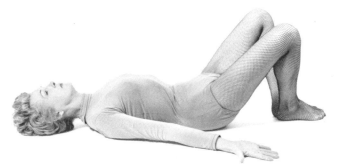

3. Before inhaling again, pull stomach in, then up under ribs. Hold. Hold. Hold. *Relax*.

✓ chart for number of times to do exercise.

12th Day	13th Day	14th Day	15th Day	16th Day	17th Day	18th Day	19th Day	20th Day	21st Day	Maintenance
5	4	4	4	4	4	5	4	5	5	5

13 *"Torso Stretch"*

TO STRETCH MUSCLES IN TORSO AND LENGTHEN WAISTLINE

PART I / "Rib Cage Stretch"

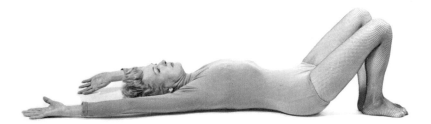

1. Lie on your back with arms extended on floor over the head, and elbows relaxed. Palms up. Bend knees. Place feet together on floor close to hips with knees slightly apart. Spine at waist is pressed to floor.

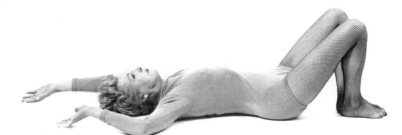

2. Keeping spine on floor, stretch up with left hand. Hold. Then relax. Next, stretch up with right hand. *Stretch* so you feel rib cage move. Keep arms as close to floor as possible.

√   chart for number of times to stretch each arm.

	1st Day	2nd Day	3rd Day	4th Day	5th Day	6th Day	7th Day	8th Day	9th Day	10th Day	11th Day
Number of times			3	3	4	4	4	4	3	3	4

PART II / "One-Legged Torso Stretch"

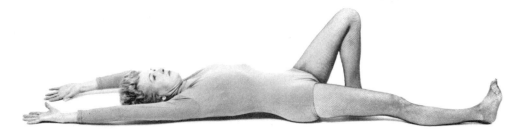

Now straighten one leg along floor. Press spine at waist to floor. Palms still up. Simultaneously stretch up with both hands and down with heel of the straight leg. *Stretch* one *long* stretch. Relax. Again press waist back, and stretch in same way.

✓ chart for number of times to stretch.

Then change legs and repeat exercise same number of times.

PART III / "Two-Legged Torso Stretch"

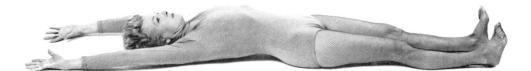

Now, both legs straight and together on floor. Spine at waist touching floor. Palms still up. Feet flexed. Stretch up with both hands and down with both heels at same time. One *long stretch*. Then relax.

✓ chart for number of times to do exercise.

12th Day	13th Day	14th Day	15th Day	16th Day	17th Day	18th Day	19th Day	20th Day	21st Day	Maintenance
4	4	4	4	3	3	3	3	4	4	4

14 *"Back Slider"*

TO FLATTEN UPPER BACK AND TO FIRM BUST

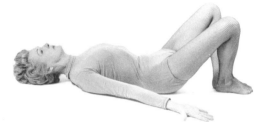

1. Lie on your back, arms at sides. Palms up. Knees bent. Feet together on floor, close to hips. Knees slightly apart. *Waist back. Ribs up. Ears up. Shoulders back and down.*

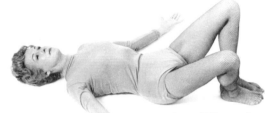

2. Keeping thumbs on floor, slowly bend your elbows and slide your arms to . . .

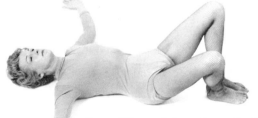

3. Shoulder level. Then stop. Check: *Waist back. Ribs up. Ears up. Shoulders back and down.*

	1st Day	2nd Day	3rd Day	4th Day	5th Day	6th Day	7th Day	8th Day	9th Day	10th Day	11t Da
Number of times			2	2	2	2	3	4	4	3	4

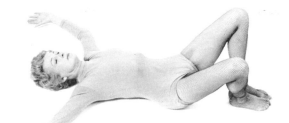

4. Keeping corrected body position, slowly slide arms on the floor . . .

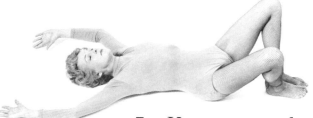

5. Up over your head, as far as you can go while keeping elbows, wrists and small of back pressed against the floor.

Now you are going to bring your arms back to the starting position in the following manner:

Keeping elbows on the floor, pull shoulders down away from ears and bring arms down 2″ (see 4). Stop. Check: *Waist back. Ribs up. Ears up. Shoulders back and down.* Then bring arms down another 2″. Stop and check body position again. Keep bringing arms down 2″ at a time until fingers reach shoulder level (see 3). Then, pulling down with your little fingers, slowly bring arms all the way down to your sides (see 1). Hold when arms are at sides and pull, pull, pull shoulders down. *Relax.*

✓ chart for number of times to do exercise.

2th Day	13th Day	14th Day	15th Day	16th Day	17th Day	18th Day	19th Day	20th Day	21st Day	Maintenance
4	2	2	2	2	2	3	2	2	4	4

15 *"Bike on Back"*

TO REDUCE LEGS AND KNEES

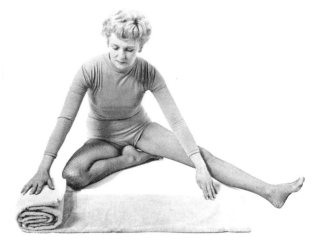

To do any exercise which requires both legs being in the air simultaneously, you must support your back. For proper back support, you will need two Turkish towels. Fold each one in half lengthwise. Roll up one folded towel. Then roll the other one around it.

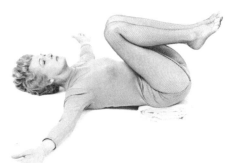

1. Lie on floor and place rolled towels under your buttocks, adjusting roll to position that will give your back the greatest support. When towel roll is in place: Extend arms to shoulder level. Palms up. Bend both knees over your chest.

	1st Day	2nd Day	3rd Day	4th Day	5th Day	6th Day	7th Day	8th Day	9th Day	10th Day	11t Da
Number of times				16	20	20	25	30	40	50	50

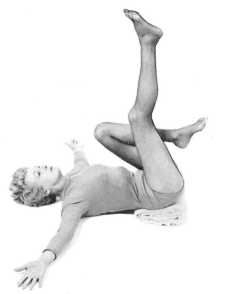

2. Straighten one leg up toward ceiling. Bring this leg toward floor, then start other leg toward ceiling as you bend and bring first leg back over chest. These movements simulate the peddling of a bicycle.

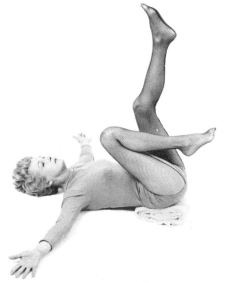

Keep your legs up over your chest; never let them drop all the way to floor. Keep feet relaxed. Do not point toes.

✓ chart for number of times to do exercise. (Count each time right leg comes up as one complete cycle.)

12th Day	13th Day	14th Day	15th Day	16th Day	17th Day	18th Day	19th Day	20th Day	21st Day	Maintenance
50	50	40	40	50	50	50	40	50	50	50

16 *"Ankle Turner"*

TO TIGHTEN MUSCLES INSIDE OF THIGHS

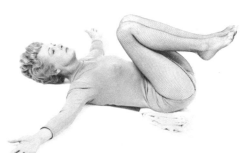

1. Lie down on floor and support your back with towels, as in Exercise 15. Extend arms to shoulder level. Palms up. Bend both knees over chest.

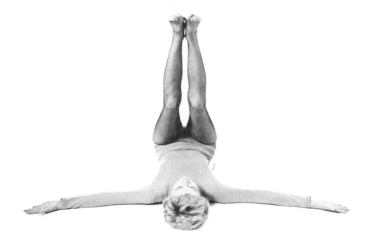

2. Extend both legs up in the air, still over your chest. Keep legs relaxed, with knees slightly bent.

	1st Day	2nd Day	3rd Day	4th Day	5th Day	6th Day	7th Day	8th Day	9th Day	10th Day	11t Da
Number of times				4	5	6	8	10	10	10	10

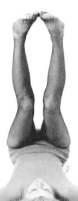

3. Turn toes in.

4. With toes turned in, spread legs wide apart. Do not force them apart more than they will comfortably go.

5. When the legs are apart, turn toes out.

6. With toes turned out, as shown, bring legs together so heels touch. Then return to position 3—ready to begin again.

√   chart for number of times to do exercise.

12th Day	13th Day	14th Day	15th Day	16th Day	17th Day	18th Day	19th Day	20th Day	21st Day	Maintenance
10	10	8	10	8	8	10	10	10	10	10

17 *"Legs Up, Wide, and Down"*

TO FIRM AND TIGHTEN FLABBY MUSCLES OF INSIDE OF THIGHS

PART I

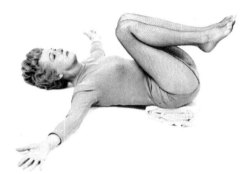

1. Lie down on floor and support your back with towels, as in Exercise 15. Extend arms to shoulder level. Palms up. Bend both knees over chest.

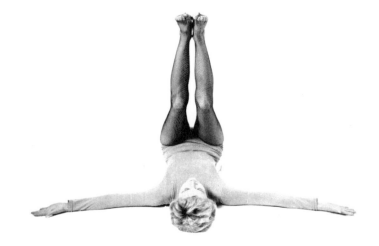

2. Now extend legs up over chest.

	1st Day	2nd Day	3rd Day	4th Day	5th Day	6th Day	7th Day	8th Day	9th Day	10th Day	11th Day
Number of times				4	5	5	5	8	10	10	10

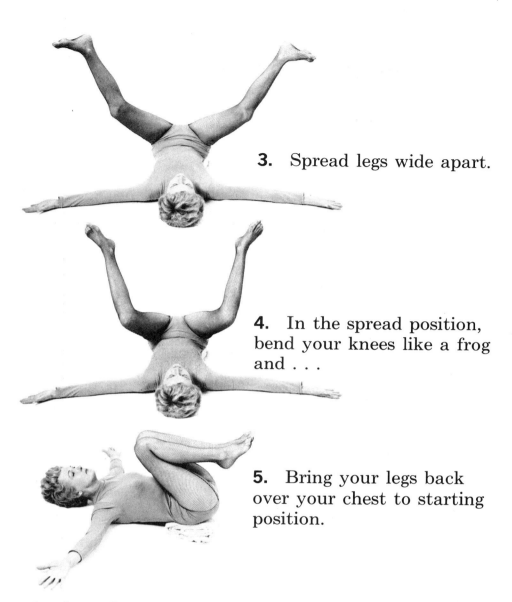

3. Spread legs wide apart.

4. In the spread position, bend your knees like a frog and . . .

5. Bring your legs back over your chest to starting position.

✓ chart for number of times to do Part I. Then do Part II same number of times.

PART II / REVERSE ACTION

From starting position, reverse entire action, going from froglike position back to starting position.

12th Day	13th Day	14th Day	15th Day	16th Day	17th Day	18th Day	19th Day	20th Day	21st Day	Maintenance
10	10	8	8	8	8	10	10	10	10	10

18 *"Frog Legs"*

FOR INSIDE OF THIGHS AND KNEES

1. Lie down on floor and support your back with towels, as in Exercise 15. Extend arms to shoulder level. Palms up. Bend both knees over chest. From this position . . .

2. Begin slowly to spread legs like a frog . . .

3. Until they are wide apart.
4. In one smooth movement, bend knees back to starting position.

√ chart for number of times to do exercise.

	1st Day	2nd Day	3rd Day	4th Day	5th Day	6th Day	7th Day	8th Day	9th Day	10th Day	11th Day
Number of times				4	5	5	5	8	10	10	10

Extra Aids for Legs

If you have a special leg problem—that is, fat thighs, drooping inner thighs, bulges at hip level, and so forth—you may need to work some additional leg exercises into your daily program. If this is the case, turn to Section II, "Five for Good Measure," where you will find those exercises which will speed up your leg reduction.

Many leg problems are caused by bad posture. Besides doing additional exercises to decrease leg measurements, you may have to become conscious of the way you are walking, sitting, and standing—all day, every day. See Section III, "Improving While Moving—All Day, Every Day."

12th Day	13th Day	14th Day	15th Day	16th Day	17th Day	18th Day	19th Day	20th Day	21st Day	Maintenance
10	10	8	8	8	8	10	10	10	10	10

19 *"Arm Push-Ups"*

TO FIRM UPPER ARMS

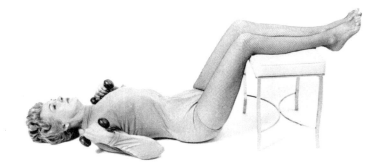

1. Lie on floor. Rest lower legs on a stool, as shown, or on a low bed, sofa or chair seat. Spine at waist should be flat on the floor. Hold a 3-pound dumbbell in each hand, with palms facing. Bend your elbows and bring arms close to your body. Keep your chin at right angle to body.

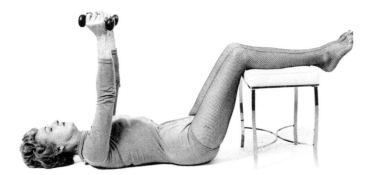

2. Straighten forearms, so hands point toward ceiling but elbows are still on floor before slowly pushing the dumbbells up until your arms are straight. Push with a nice, smooth motion. No jerking. No snapping of elbows.

	1st Day	2nd Day	3rd Day	4th Day	5th Day	6th Day	7th Day	8th Day	9th Day	10th Day	11th Day
Number of times					8	8	10	10	12	12	14

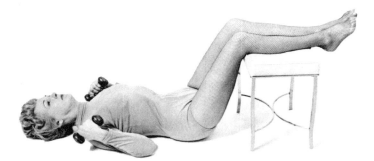

3. Slowly bring the dumbbells straight down again, bending elbows as arms move down.

√   chart for number of times to do exercise.

This exercise, and the following three, can be done without weights, but the arm muscles can be toned more quickly if 3-pound dumbbells are used (a man may use 5-pound dumbbells, but no heavier). (See Weights, page 6.)

2th Day	13th Day	14th Day	15th Day	16th Day	17th Day	18th Day	19th Day	20th Day	21st Day	Maintenance
16	16	18	20	20	18	20	20	20	20	20

20 *"Breast Stroke"*

TO FIRM ENTIRE ARM AND BUST

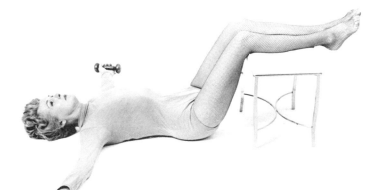

1. Lie on floor with lower legs resting on stool. *Waist back. Ears up.* Arms extended on floor, shoulder level. Backs of hands resting on floor, with a 3-pound dumbbell in each hand.

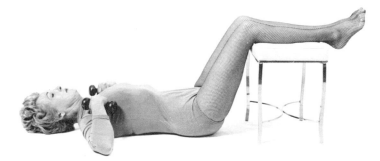

2. Bend elbows and bring dumbbells toward shoulders, keeping elbows, upper arms and shoulders on floor.

	1st Day	2nd Day	3rd Day	4th Day	5th Day	6th Day	7th Day	8th Day	9th Day	10th Day	11th Day
Number of times				4	5	6	8	8	8	10

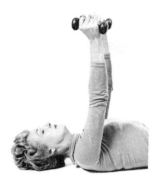 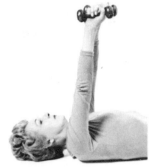 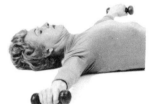

3. Straighten arms up toward ceiling, palms facing each other.

4. Turn palms out, and . . .

5. Slowly lower arms to floor.

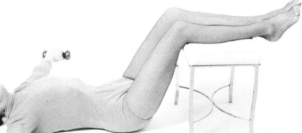 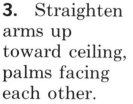

6. With dumbbells resting on floor, turn hands to . . .

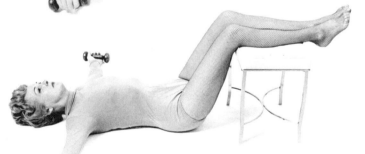

7. Palms-up position—ready to begin again.

√ chart for number of times to do exercise.

12th Day	13th Day	14th Day	15th Day	16th Day	17th Day	18th Day	19th Day	20th Day	21st Day	Maintenance
10	10	10	10	10	8	10	10	10	10	10

21 "Slow-Motion Clap"

TO FIRM CHEST MUSCLES AND BUST

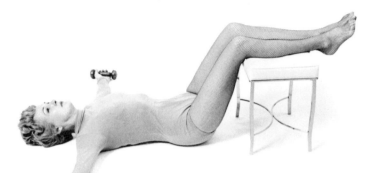

1. Lie on floor with lower legs resting on stool. *Waist back. Ears up.* Arms extended on floor, shoulder level. Backs of hands resting on floor, with a 3-pound dumbbell in each hand.

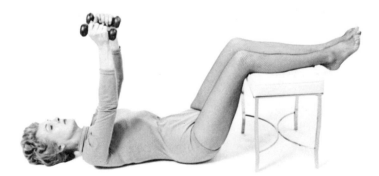

2. Keeping arms straight, slowly raise them up over chest, until . . .

	1st Day	2nd Day	3rd Day	4th Day	5th Day	6th Day	7th Day	8th Day	9th Day	10th Day	11th Da
Number of times					5	5	6	8	8	8	1(

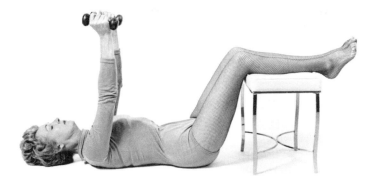

3. Dumbbells almost meet in center.

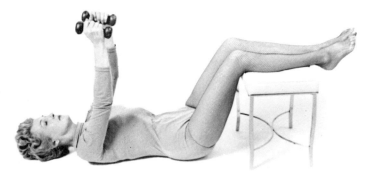

4. Still keeping arms straight, *slowly* lower them, until . . .

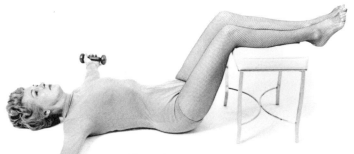

5. Backs of hands again touch the floor.

✓ chart for number of times to do exercise.

th ay	13th Day	14th Day	15th Day	16th Day	17th Day	18th Day	19th Day	20th Day	21st Day	Maintenance
0	10	10	10	10	8	10	10	10	10	10

22 *"Bicep-Firmer"*

TO FIRM FRONT OF UPPER ARMS

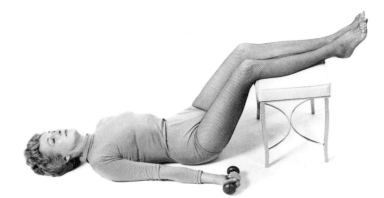

1. Lie on floor with lower legs resting on stool. *Waist back. Ears up.* Arms on floor, at your sides, close to the body. Backs of hands resting on floor, with a 3-pound dumbbell in each hand.

	1st Day	2nd Day	3rd Day	4th Day	5th Day	6th Day	7th Day	8th Day	9th Day	10th Day	11th Day
Number of times					8	10	10	10	12	12	14

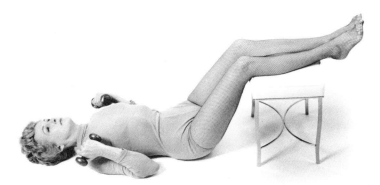

2. Slowly bend your elbows, keeping them on floor. Bring dumbbells to your shoulders.

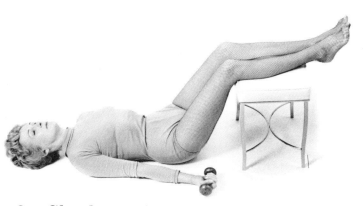

3. Slowly straighten arms and lower dumbbells back down to the floor to the starting position.

✓ chart for number of times to do exercise.

2th Day	13th Day	14th Day	15th Day	16th Day	17th Day	18th Day	19th Day	20th Day	21st Day	Maintenance
6	16	18	20	20	18	20	20	20	20	20

23 *"Leg Circles"*

TO REDUCE THIGHS

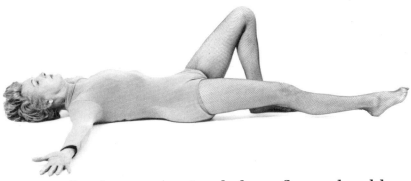

1. Lie on your back, arms extended on floor, shoulder level. Palms up. Bend left leg and place foot on floor, close to hips. Keep right leg straight. You are going to make circles with the straight leg.

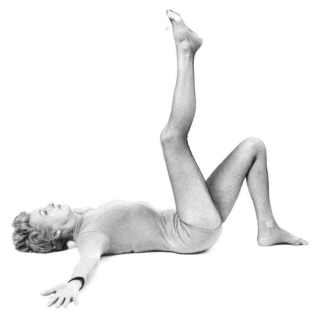

2. Raise straightened leg toward ceiling.

	1st Day	2nd Day	3rd Day	4th Day	5th Day	6th Day	7th Day	8th Day	9th Day	10th Day	11th Day
Number of times						8	9	12	12	12	

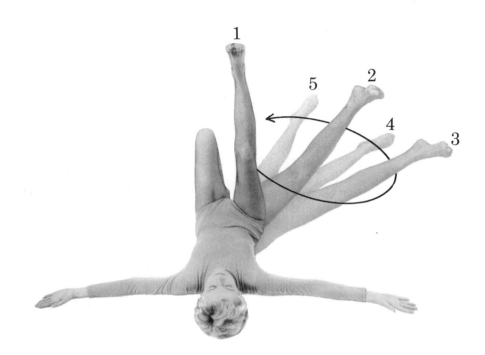

3. Then make a sweeping circle with it, out away from body, then down toward floor, in toward your bent left leg. (Do not touch circling leg to floor.) Then bring it straight up toward ceiling, and circle again.

✓ chart for number of times to circle.

4. Now bend the right leg and straighten the left leg, and do same number of circles with left leg.

5. Then do reverse circles with each leg, same number of times.

Remember to keep the non-circling leg bent. This prevents straining back muscles.

2th Day	13th Day	14th Day	15th Day	16th Day	17th Day	18th Day	19th Day	20th Day	21st Day	Maintenance
15	12	12	12	15	15	12	15	15	15	15

24 *"Upsy-Downsy"*

TO STRENGTHEN AND FLATTEN ABDOMEN

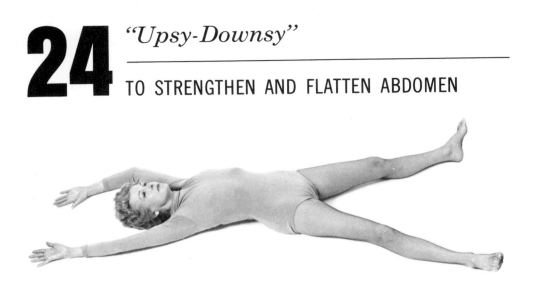

1. Lie on your back, arms extended over your head on the floor. Palms up. Legs straight and apart. Keep knees slightly bent.

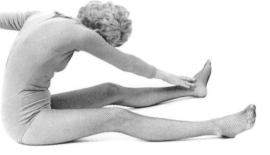

2. Now in a continuous motion, swing arms up, come to a sitting position, bend forward and bring right hand toward left foot. Don't force the bend. Be loose and relaxed. Left arm is extended out back.

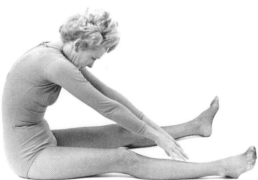

3. Bring hands together between legs.

	1st Day	2nd Day	3rd Day	4th Day	5th Day	6th Day	7th Day	8th Day	9th Day	10th Day	11th Day
Number of times								4	4	6	6

4. Slowly lower yourself back to the floor, pulling stomach in all the way down.

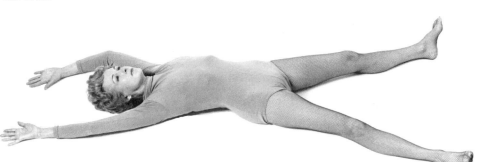

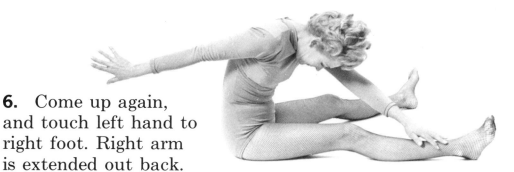

5. As arms go back to the floor, pull stomach in and up under ribs.

6. Come up again, and touch left hand to right foot. Right arm is extended out back.

✓ chart for number of times to do exercise, each time alternating arm and leg.

If you have difficulty in bringing yourself up for the first time from position 1, start the exercise by going down first (from position 3). Generally people work up momentum and can come up the next time from the lying-down position.

2th Day	13th Day	14th Day	15th Day	16th Day	17th Day	18th Day	19th Day	20th Day	21st Day	Maintenance
6	8	8	8	8	8	8	8	8	8	8

25 "Hip Walk"

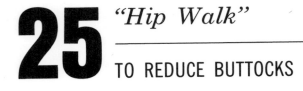

TO REDUCE BUTTOCKS

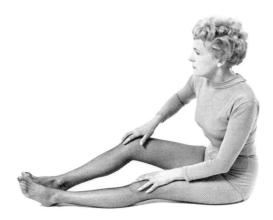

1. Sit on the floor, legs straight out in front, hands resting on knees. Now "walk" forward on your hips. Lift your right hip and leg and slide right foot forward. Then lift left hip and leg and move that foot forward. Let knees bend slightly as you lift legs. Take 10 forward "steps" on buttocks.

	1st Day	2nd Day	3rd Day	4th Day	5th Day	6th Day	7th Day	8th Day	9th Day	10th Day	11th Day
Number of times									2	2	2

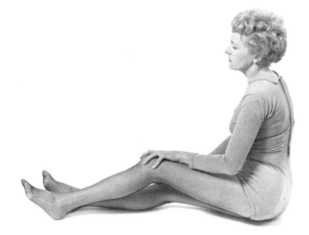

2. Now "walk" backward. Lift right hip, left hip. Always walk same number of "steps" backward as you go forward.

✓ chart for number of times to take 10 "steps" forward and 10 "steps" backward.

2th Day	13th Day	14th Day	15th Day	16th Day	17th Day	18th Day	19th Day	20th Day	21st Day	Maintenance
3	3	4	5	5	4	5	4	5	5	5

26 *"Hip Roll"*
FOR REDUCING LOWER HIPS AND OUTSIDE OF TOP OF THIGHS

1. Sit on the floor, legs straight, feet together, heels on floor, arms extended slightly behind body, palms on the floor.

2. Keeping legs straight, roll over onto your left hip and catch your weight on your left hand. Stretch right arm up over your head. Really *stretch* that arm. Keep heels on floor.

	1st Day	2nd Day	3rd Day	4th Day	5th Day	6th Day	7th Day	8th Day	9th Day	10th Day	11th Day
Number of times									8	16	20

3. Continuing to keep legs straight, roll over onto right hip. Catch weight on right hand. Stretch left arm up over your head.

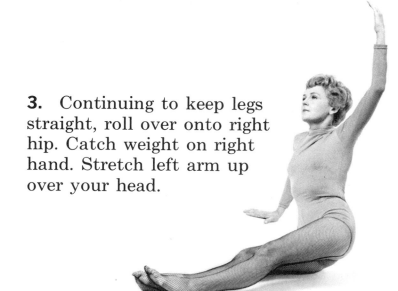

√   chart for number of times to do exercise.

NOTE: Rolling the body on the floor, of itself, doesn't break up fat. Fat is broken up by the contracting of muscles in conjunction with the relaxing of opposite muscles.

2th Day	13th Day	14th Day	15th Day	16th Day	17th Day	18th Day	19th Day	20th Day	21st Day	Maintenance
20	20	26	26	26	26	24	24	26	26	26

27

"Press the Ball"

TO FIRM AND TIGHTEN ARMS AND BUST

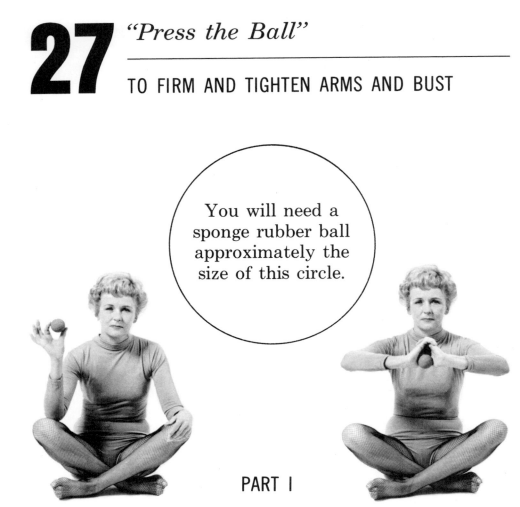

You will need a sponge rubber ball approximately the size of this circle.

PART I

Sit on a chair, or tailor-fashion on floor, as shown.

Bend your arms and bring elbows to chest height, with hands about 8″ away from body. Place ball between your palms, resting it on the heels of your hands, with fingers interlocked.

Press the heels of your hands against the ball for the count of 5. Relax the pressure.

✓ chart for number of times to do exercise.

	1st Day	2nd Day	3rd Day	4th Day	5th Day	6th Day	7th Day	8th Day	9th Day	10th Day	11th Day
Number of times										5	8

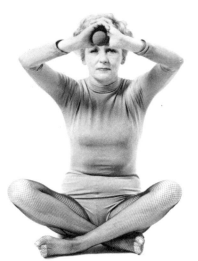

PART II

Raise hands to forehead level. Press the ball between heels of interlocked hands and hold pressure for count of 5. Then relax.

√ chart for number of times to do exercise.

PART III

Bring arms behind back, at hip level. Press the ball between heels of interlocked hands and hold pressure for count of 5. Then relax.

√ chart for number of times to do exercise.

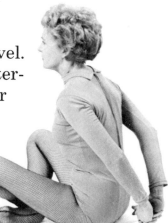

12th Day	13th Day	14th Day	15th Day	16th Day	17th Day	18th Day	19th Day	20th Day	21st Day	Maintenance
10	10	10	8	8	8	10	10	10	10	10

28 *"The Sitting Bends"*
FOR THE WAIST, UPPER HIPS, UPPER BACK AND CHEST

1. Sit on the floor, legs apart, knees relaxed, not stiff. Arms up over your head. Clasp hands and turn palms up toward ceiling.

2. Bend toward your right foot. Keep knees relaxed. Don't force the bend. Bend only as far as the body wants to go.

3. Come back up. Bring arms behind ears. Pull stomach in. Chest up.

	1st Day	2nd Day	3rd Day	4th Day	5th Day	6th Day	7th Day	8th Day	9th Day	10th Day	11t Da
Number of times											

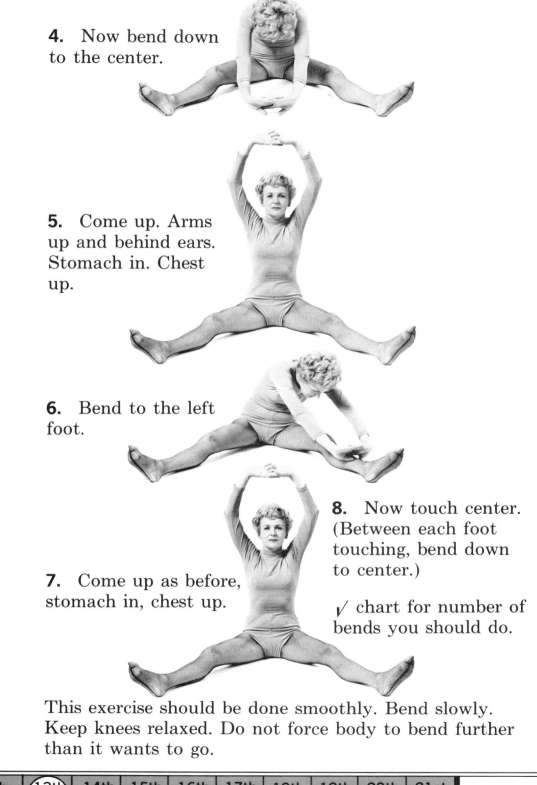

4. Now bend down to the center.

5. Come up. Arms up and behind ears. Stomach in. Chest up.

6. Bend to the left foot.

7. Come up as before, stomach in, chest up.

8. Now touch center. (Between each foot touching, bend down to center.)

√ chart for number of bends you should do.

This exercise should be done smoothly. Bend slowly. Keep knees relaxed. Do not force body to bend further than it wants to go.

2th ʲay	13th Day	14th Day	15th Day	16th Day	17th Day	18th Day	19th Day	20th Day	21st Day	Maintenance
8	8	12	12	14	16	14	16	16		16

29

"Hand-to-Toe Bends"

TO REDUCE WAISTLINE AND UPPER HIPS

1. Sit on the floor, legs apart, knees relaxed. Arms out, shoulder level. Palms up. *Waist back. Ribs up. Ears up.*

2. Bend toward the left and bring the right hand toward left foot loose and relaxed. Left arm is extended out back.

Don't force the bending. Go only as far as the body wants to go.

3. Return to position 1. Then bend left hand to right foot loose and relaxed. Right arm is extended out back. Again return to position 1.

✓ chart for number of times to do exercise.

	1st Day	2nd Day	3rd Day	4th Day	5th Day	6th Day	7th Day	8th Day	9th Day	10th Day	11 Da
Number of times											

30

"Clasped-Hands Push-Backs"

TO FLATTEN UPPER BACK

Sit on a stool with feet flat on the floor. Push your spine at the waistline out back. Raise both arms over your head just in front of your ears. Clasp hands and turn palms up. Keeping hands clasped in this manner, push both arms so they go behind your ears. Relax.

√ chart for number of times to move arms back and forth.

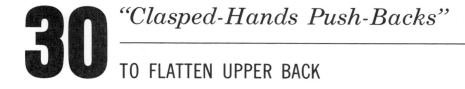

Don't lean back. Don't let your head come forward. Just move those arms.

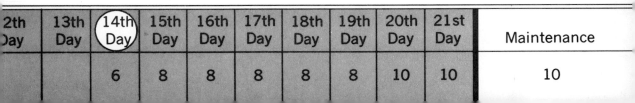

2th Day	13th Day	14th Day	15th Day	16th Day	17th Day	18th Day	19th Day	20th Day	21st Day	Maintenance
		6	8	8	8	8	8	10	10	10

31 "Standing Stretch"

TO STRETCH THE TORSO, ABDOMEN, UPPER HIPS AND BACK / PART I

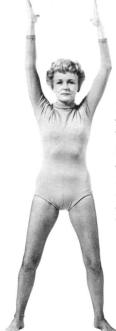

1. Stand with legs apart, for balance. Bend your knees, tuck your hips under. (Tuck those hips under like a puppy whose rump is about to be smacked.) Raise both arms up over your head, palms facing each other.

2. Keeping the "tucked" position, stretch up toward the ceiling with the right hand (which almost automatically will bring the left arm into an angled position). Then stretch up with the left hand. Stretch so your rib cage moves up and your hips remain stationary. Stretch with loose and relaxed motions, in rhythm.

√   chart for number of times to do exercise.

	1st Day	2nd Day	3rd Day	4th Day	5th Day	6th Day	7th Day	8th Day	9th Day	10th Day	11t Da
Number of times											

"Bending Stretch"
FOR THE WAIST AND UPPER HIPS / PART II

1.   Stand with legs apart. Keep hips "tucked" under.
Keep knees bent. Place hands on hips just below the waist.

2.   Bend to the right (with a "bouncy" movement)
3 times; do not come up all the way between "bounces."
Keep the head relaxed. Let it go to the right with the
body. Keep both feet firmly planted on ground.

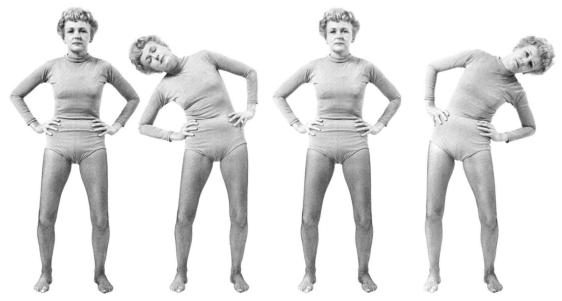

3.   Then come back up and resume position 1.

4.   Now "bounce" to the left 3 times. Head relaxed.
Let it go with the body. Then come back up and resume
position 1.

✓   chart for number of times to do exercise. Count
left and right bend as 1.

> NOTE: In all bending exercises, go only as far
> as the muscles give. Gradually they will give
> more and you will bend further.

12th Day	13th Day	14th Day	15th Day	16th Day	17th Day	18th Day	19th Day	20th Day	21st Day		ntenance
			6		8	8	8	10	10		10

32 "The Highland Fling"

TO STRAIGHTEN UPPER BACK AND FIRM CHEST MUSCLES AND BUST / PART I

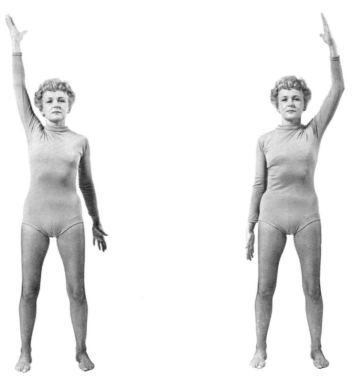

1. Stand with feet apart, knees bent, hips "tucked" under. *Right* arm extended *up* over the head. *Left* arm *down*. Palms facing in toward body. Keep both arms parallel to body and rhythmically "chop" the air with your arms. First both arms go back, then they come forward slightly. "Chop" air 5 times with arms in this position.

2. Now reverse arm positions. *Left* arm *up*. *Right* arm *down*. Again push arms back and forth 5 times.

✓ chart for number of times to change arm positions.

	1st Day	2nd Day	3rd Day	4th Day	5th Day	6th Day	7th Day	8th Day	9th Day	10th Day	11t Da
Number of times											

"Curved-Arm Stretch"
FOR THE WAIST, UPPER HIPS AND UPPER BACK / PART II

1. Stand with feet apart, knees bent, hips "tucked" under. Raise arms to shoulder level. Palms up.

2. Keeping knees bent, "bounce" body to the left 3 times. As you bend, curve right arm over the head. Turn palm of left hand and hold it against left thigh to give support to body as you "bounce."

3. Return to starting position. Now: *Waist back. Ribs up. Ears up.* Palms up.

4. Next, bend body to the right 3 times. This time, left hand over the head, right hand to thigh.

√ chart for number of times to do exercise. Count left and right bend as 1.

12th Day	13th Day	14th Day	15th Day	16th Day	17th Day	18th Day	19th Day	20th Day	21st Day	Maintenance
					4	4	4	5	6	6

33 "The Toe-Touchers' Squat"

FOR THE WAIST, HIPS, THIGHS, BACK AND CHEST

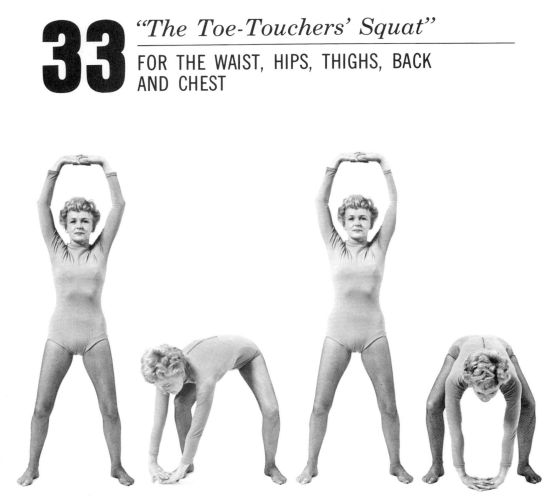

1. Stand with feet apart. Bend knees and "tuck" hips under. Raise both arms over your head. Clasp your hands and turn palms up toward the ceiling.

2. Bending knees deeply, touch clasped hands to toes of right foot.

3. Come up, hands back over your head.

4. Bending knees deeply, touch hands between your feet.

	1st Day	2nd Day	3rd Day	4th Day	5th Day	6th Day	7th Day	8th Day	9th Day	10th Day	11th Day
Number of times											

5. Come up, hands back over your head.

6. Bending knees deeply, touch clasped hands to toes of left foot.

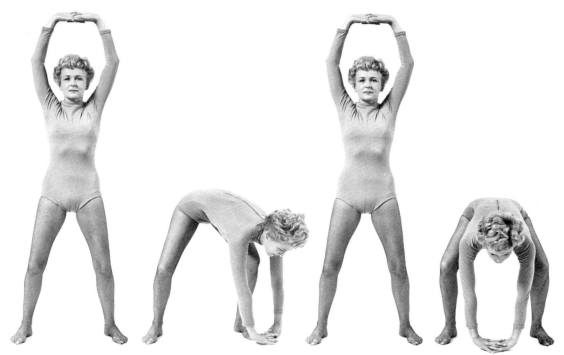

7. Come up, hands back up over your head.

8. Now, bending knees deeply, touch hands between your feet. (Between each toe-touching, bend down to center.)

√ chart for total number of bends.

NOTE: NEVER, NEVER try to touch floor from a standing position without BENDING YOUR KNEES. If you do, you'll run the risk of hurting your back.

12th Day	13th Day	14th Day	15th Day	16th Day	17th Day	18th Day	19th Day	20th Day	21st Day	Maintenance
							8	12	16	16

34 *"The Octopus"*
TO STRAIGHTEN UPPER BACK, LIFT CHEST AND FIRM BUST AND UPPER ARMS

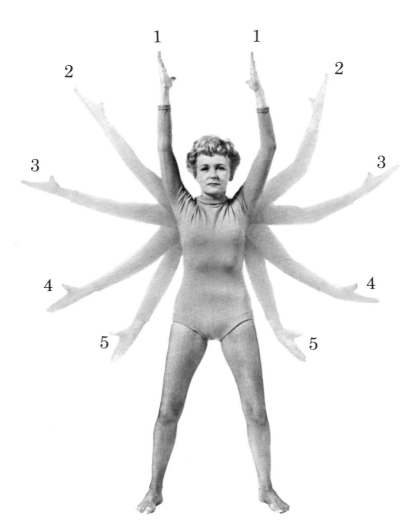

Stand with feet apart. Bend knees and "tuck" hips under.

(Arm positions are illustrated above. Note that elbows are relaxed but fairly straight.)

	1st Day	2nd Day	3rd Day	4th Day	5th Day	6th Day	7th Day	8th Day	9th Day	10th Day	11th Day
Number of times											

1. Raise arms straight up over your head, with palms facing each other. (See arm position marked 1.)
With a rhythmic motion, push both arms back of ears, then bring them forward to their starting position. Keep head still as you rock arms back and forth. Keep chin at right angle to your neck. Rock arms back and forth 5 times.

2. Now drop arms halfway to shoulder. (See arm position marked 2.) Palms face up. Keeping arms at this level, rock arms back and forth 5 times.

3. Now drop arms to shoulder level. (See arm position marked 3.) Palms face up. Rock arms back and forth at this level 5 times.

4. Now drop arms halfway between hips and shoulders. (See arm position marked 4.) Palms face up. Rock arms back and forth at this level 5 times.

5. Next, drop arms to hip level. Palms face forward. Rock arms back and forth at this level 5 times.

✓ chart for number of times to do entire exercise.

12th Day	13th Day	14th Day	15th Day	16th Day	17th Day	18th Day	19th Day	20th Day	21st Day	Maintenance
								1	2	2

35 *"Standing Back-Slider"*

TO FLATTEN UPPER BACK

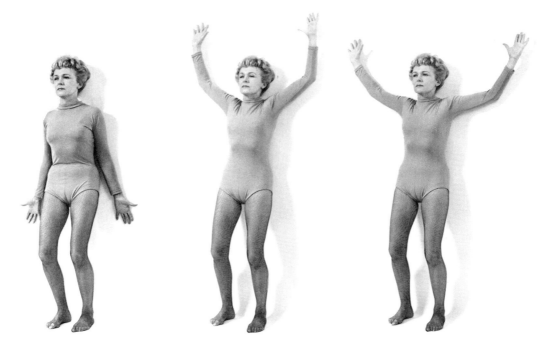

1. Stand against a wall with your feet parallel, about 4″ apart and 4″ away from wall, toes pointing straight ahead. Arms at your sides and pressed against the wall, palms out. Bend knees and slide down wall until the spine at the waist touches the wall.

2. Raise arms above head and try to touch wall with them, but don't pull spine away from wall to do so.

3. Pull shoulders down away from your ears and bring arms down about 2″. Hold.

	1st Day	2nd Day	3rd Day	4th Day	5th Day	6th Day	7th Day	8th Day	9th Day	10th Day	11th Day
Number of times											

4. Keeping shoulders pulled down, spine at wall, bring arms down a couple more inches. As arms go down, gradually straighten them, keeping them against wall.

5. Again, shoulders and spine at wall, pull shoulders down and bring arms gradually lower.

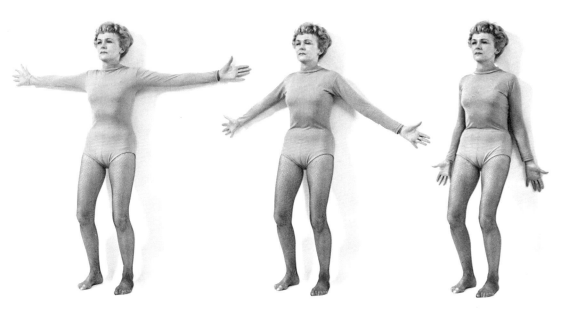

6. Now pull down with your little fingers and bring arms all the way down to your sides. Chin parallel with floor. *Shoulders back and down.* HOLD. *Relax.*

✓ chart for number of times to do exercise.

You've done a form of this exercise on the floor. It is more difficult to do while standing—gravity is pulling at you. But don't be discouraged. As your muscles are toned (and toning can be accelerated by doing more of Exercise 14), you'll be able to get those arms flat against the wall along with your spine.

2th Day	13th Day	14th Day	15th Day	16th Day	17th Day	18th Day	19th Day	20th Day	21st Day	Maintenance
									2	2

SECTION II

FIVE FOR GOOD MEASURE

Now that you've reached the Maintenance level of your 21-Day Shape-Up Program, the time has come for you to take a hard critical look at yourself. If your body is toning up uniformly with the maintenance program, you will not need to add any of the exercises in this section. If, however, you find you have areas which are not shaping up as quickly as others, this is the time for you to personalize the maintenance program by adding some specific area exercises to it. In this way, within the limits of your bone structure, you can literally sculpture your body to the contour you want.

Within the "Five for Good Measure" section you will find units of five specific exercises each for arms, upper back, abdomen, upper hips, buttocks and thighs, outside of thighs, inside of thighs—and extra beautification and corrective exercises for posture, knees, ankles, knockknees and bowlegs. Within each unit you will find how to work these exercises into your daily program.

Some exercises in this section require a rubber ball, dumbbells or ankle weights. The rubber ball and dumbbells are pictured in use in the exercises that call for them. The ankle weights are shown wrapped around the ankles for exercises where they are to be worn. (For example, see Exercise 57.) For explanation of why these things are used, see Equipment, page 6.

Once all parts of your body become contoured to their perfect proportions, you still must continue doing extra exercises for your problem spots, for they were larger or flabbier to begin with, and thus were harder for you to reduce and firm—and if you do gain weight, these will *always* be your problem spots.

36 *"Five for Good Measure"*

ARMS

To hasten firming and shaping of upper arms, increase the number of times you do Exercise 34 to 4 times, and add all five of the arm exercises in this unit to your daily program. *Work with dumbbells only in the exercises that specifically call for them.*

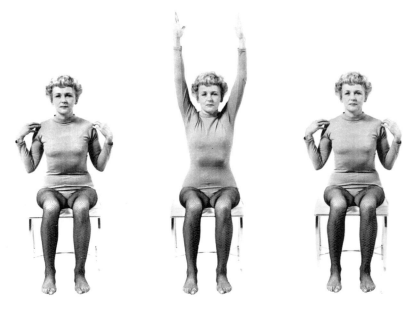

1. Sit on a stool, with feet flat on the floor. Bend elbows and bring fingertips to shoulders.

2. Straighten arms up over your head.

3. Bring fingertips down to shoulders again, elbows close to body.

Repeat exercise until arms get tired.

Do the movements fast and loose. Do not tense your arms.

37 "Five for Good Measure"

ARMS

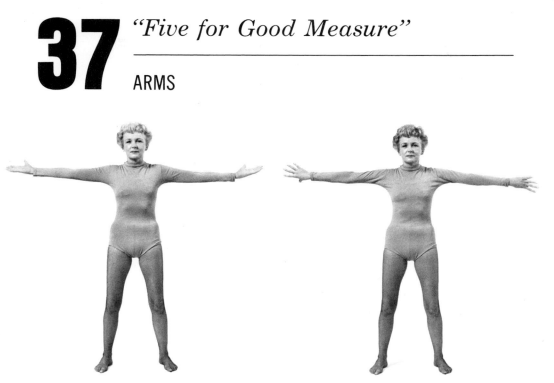

1. Stand with knees slightly bent, hips "tucked" under. Arms extended at shoulder level. Palms up. **2.** Twist your arms by turning thumbs down and back. Hold. **3.** Reverse this movement so the palms are facing up again.

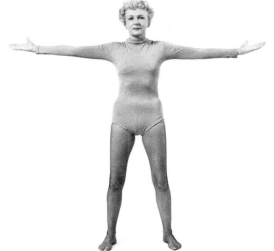

Repeat exercise until arms get tired.

38 *"Five for Good Measure"*

ARMS

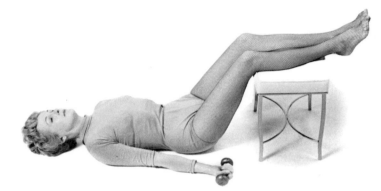

1. Lie on floor with legs resting on stool. *Waist back. Ears up.* Arms are on the floor, close to your body. Backs of hands rest on floor, with a 3-pound dumbbell in each hand (a man may use 5-pound dumbbells, but no heavier).

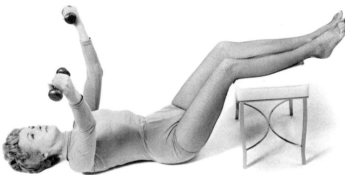

2. Slowly straighten arms up toward ceiling to shoulder level.

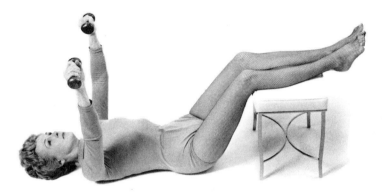

3. Turn hands so palms face your feet.

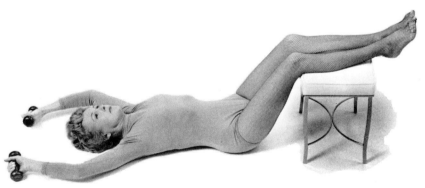

4. Slowly lower arms back over your head to the floor, until backs of hands rest on floor.

5. Then reverse action: Slowly bring arms up toward ceiling to shoulder level. Turn hands so that backs of hands face the feet. Slowly lower arms forward to the floor.

Do exercise 10 times.

39 *"Five for Good Measure"*

ARMS

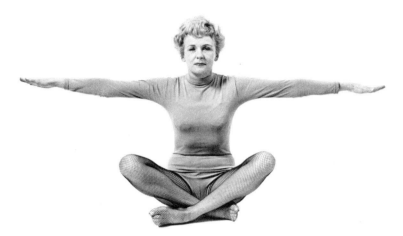

1. Sit on a stool, with feet flat on the floor, or on the floor, tailor-fashion. Bring arms out to shoulder level. Palms down.

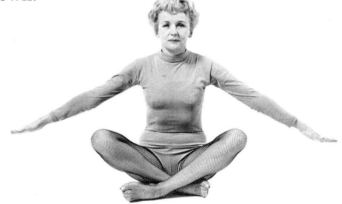

2. Now tense your arms and slowly lower them to sides of your body. Keep arms tensed all the way down.

Now relax arms, then bring them loosely back up to shoulder level.

Do exercise 10 times.

40 "Five for Good Measure"

ARMS

1. Sit on a stool, with feet flat on the floor, or on the floor, tailor-fashion. Bring arms out to shoulder level. Palms down.

2. Slowly bend elbows and with tensed arms bring fingers to chest.

3. Straighten arms back out. When arm is fully extended, tense arms so the underneath of upper arm pulls up.

Do exercise 10 times.

41 *"Five for Good Measure"*

UPPER BACK

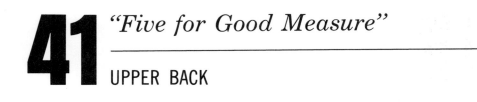

To hasten the reduction of fat around the upper back, do more than the suggested Maintenance level of Exercises 4, 14, 28, 32, 34 and 35. In addition, do at least two exercises (41 and 44) from this unit, though all five can be done if desired.

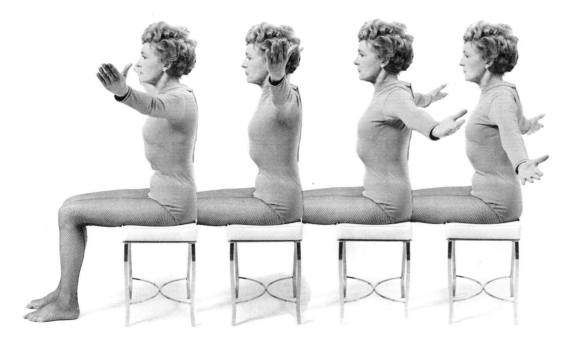

Sit on a stool with feet flat on the floor (or sit tailor-fashion on floor). Bring arms out to shoulder level. Palms up. Now move arms in small circles, up, back and down.

Do exercise 10 times.

42 *"Five for Good Measure"*

UPPER BACK

1

2

4

3

1. Stand with hips "tucked" under. Raise arms above your head. Clasp hands and turn palms up.

2. Now circle arms to the right . . .

3. Then down in front of body . . .

4. Then up to the left . . . and over your head again.

Go around and around, with arms loose and relaxed.

Do 20 times; then reverse circle and do 20 times more.

43 *"Five for Good Measure"*

UPPER BACK

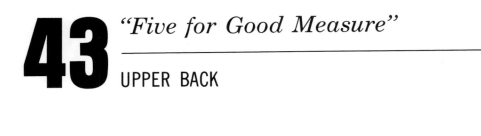

1. Lie on the floor on your back, with legs wide apart and fingertips on shoulders.

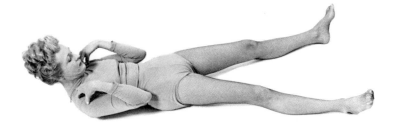

2. Lift head off the floor and look down at your toes.

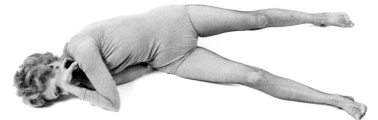

3. Roll across your upper back, bringing your left elbow over your body and as close to the floor on the right side as you can. Then roll over to the other side, bringing the right elbow to the floor on the left side. Over and back. Keep your feet on the floor.

Do exercise 20 times.

44 *"Five for Good Measure"*

UPPER BACK

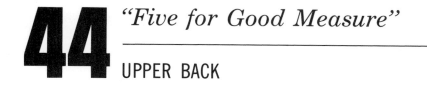

1. Lie down on the floor on your side, with both arms up over your head. Rest head on underneath arm. Palms are facing floor. Underneath leg is bent; top leg is straight.

2. Swing the top arm behind you. Keep it parallel to your body. At the same time swing your top leg, with knee slightly bent, up toward your chest.

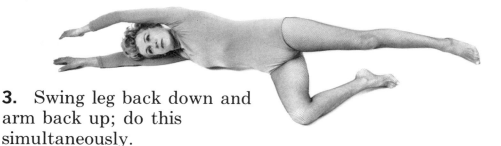

3. Swing leg back down and arm back up; do this simultaneously.

Do exercise 15 times. Then roll over and do exercise 15 times on other side.

45 *"Five for Good Measure"*

UPPER BACK

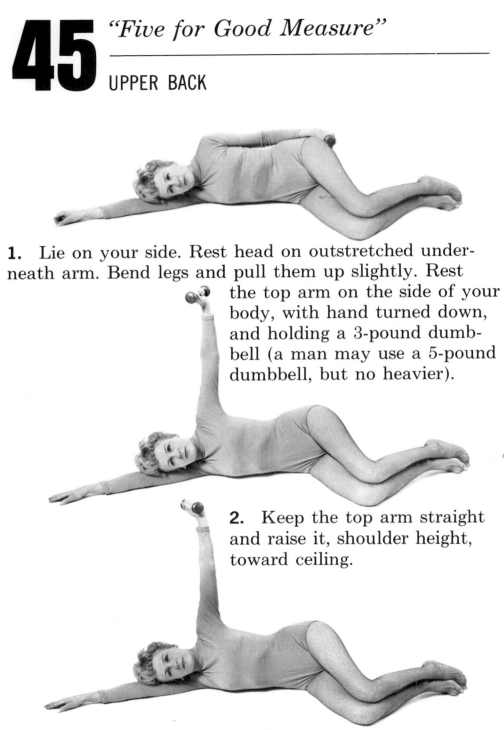

1. Lie on your side. Rest head on outstretched underneath arm. Bend legs and pull them up slightly. Rest the top arm on the side of your body, with hand turned down, and holding a 3-pound dumbbell (a man may use a 5-pound dumbbell, but no heavier).

2. Keep the top arm straight and raise it, shoulder height, toward ceiling.

3. Turn arm so palm of hand is turned toward head.

4. Lower dumbbell to floor above head. Keep arm as straight as possible.

5. Raise arm back up, shoulder height, keeping palm toward head.

6. Turn hand so palm faces feet and lower arm down to your body.

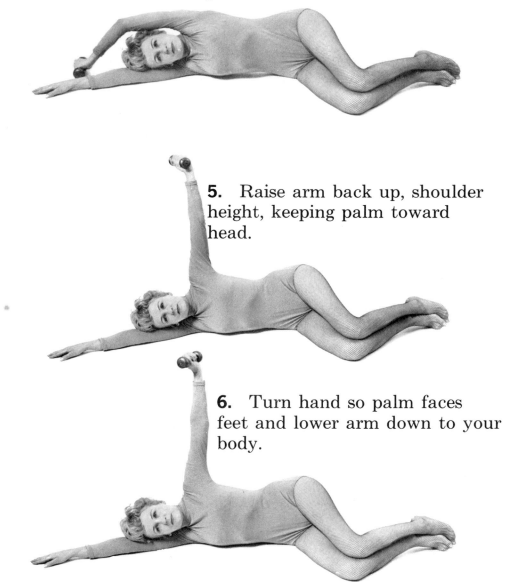

Do exercise 5 times; then roll over and repeat on the other side. Gradually try to increase entire exercise to 10 times.

46 *"Five for Good Measure"*

ABDOMEN

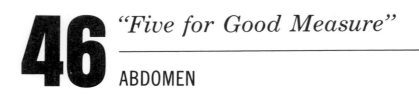

To strengthen the abdominal muscles more quickly, keep pulling the abdomen in and up all day long. Increase the number of times you do Exercises 11, 12 and 24 beyond those suggested for Maintenance level. In addition, add all five of the abdomen exercises in this unit to your daily program.

1. Stand against a wall with your feet parallel, about 4″ apart and 4″ away from wall, toes pointing straight ahead. Bend knees and slide down wall until the spine at the waist touches the wall.

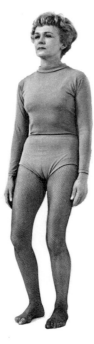

2. Separate knees further without moving feet. Pull *waist back* against wall, *rib cage up* away from hips, *ears up* away from shoulders. *Shoulders* should be *back and down,* away from ears.

3. Pull stomach in tight. Hold. Pull stomach in more. Hold. Pull stomach in still more. Hold.

Relax.

Do exercise 8 times.

47 *"Five for Good Measure"*

ABDOMEN

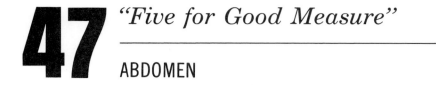

1. Lie down on the floor with your feet on a stool or bed. Extend arms over your head. Palms up.

2. Now swing the arms up, and then toward knees, to help propel you . . .

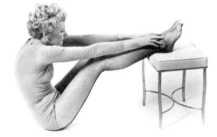

3. To a sitting position, and try to touch toes with outstretched hands.

4. Go back down slowly, pulling stomach in all the way down.

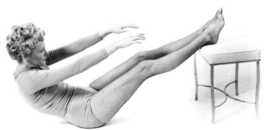

5. When arms are on the floor over your head, pull stomach in and up under ribs.

Do exercise 5 times.

48 *"Five for Good Measure"*

ABDOMEN

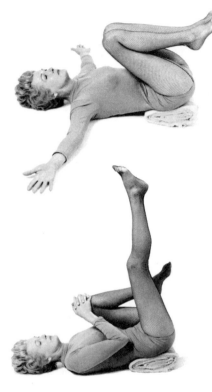

1. Lie down on the floor, with two Turkish towels folded (see Exercise 15) and placed under your lower hips. Arms extended, shoulder level. Palms up. Bend both knees over your chest.

2. Clasp hands around left knee and pull the leg toward your chest. Straighten right leg up toward the ceiling, and pulling stomach in tight, slowly lower it down toward the floor.

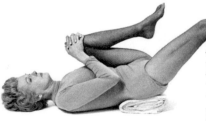

3. Lower the leg only down to hip level—never to the floor. Hold. Return to starting position. Now raise left leg and repeat.

Do complete exercise 8 times.

49

"Five for Good Measure"

ABDOMEN

1. Lie down on the floor, knees bent and slightly apart, feet together on the floor, and close to your hips. Arms extended, shoulder level. Elbows bent slightly. Palms up.

2. Slowly lift spine off the floor, one vertebra at a time, starting with the coccyx (the base of the spine). When you are up as far as you can go, press arms back against the floor.

3. Keep pressing as you slowly lower your spine back down. As you come down, pull stomach in (down toward the floor).

4. Keep hips raised until you lower small of back to floor, then bring hips down.

Do exercise 5 times.

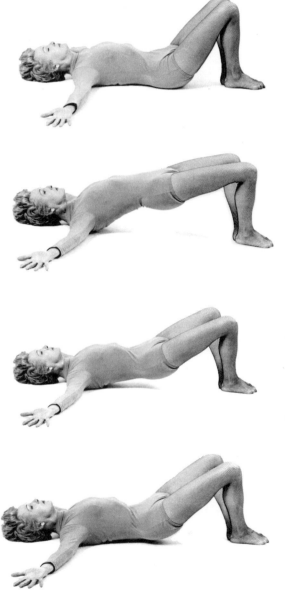

50 "Five for Good Measure"

ABDOMEN

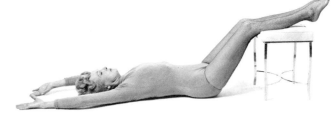

1. Lie down on the floor with lower legs resting on a stool. Arms over the head on the floor. Palms up.

2. Slowly lift spine off the floor, one vertebra at a time, starting with the coccyx (the base of the spine). Up, up, up.

3. When you are up, stretch from the tip of your fingers to the tip of your toes.

4. Then come down slowly, one vertebra at a time, starting at the top. As you come down, pull stomach in (down toward the floor). Keep hips raised until you lower small of back to floor, then bring hips down.

Do exercise 5 times.

51 *"Five for Good Measure"*

UPPER HIPS

To hasten the reduction of fat around the upper hips, you will need to do more stretching and bending to the side. Do at least Exercises 51, 53 and 54 (though it would not hurt to do all upper-hip exercises) and do more than the suggested Maintenance level of Exercises 4, 5, 7, 8 and 13.

1. Sit on your right hip, with right leg bent under. Right arm is stretched out from shoulder and hand is flat on the floor. Top leg is straight and slightly forward.

2. Now raise up on your right knee and stretch the left arm over your body. Stretch 3 times with a "bouncy" movement.

3. Now sit back down on your hips. Bring right hand to left foot. Stretch left arm behind back. Bend forward with a "bouncy" movement 3 times.

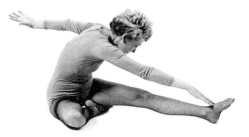

Do exercise 8 times. Then do exercise 8 times sitting on left hip.

52 *"Five for Good Measure"*

UPPER HIPS

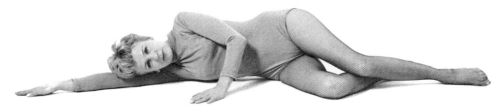

1. Lie on your side, in slight semicircle position, with head resting on underneath outstretched arm. Place hand of other arm on floor in front of chest, for support. Bend your underneath leg and keep it bent throughout exercise.

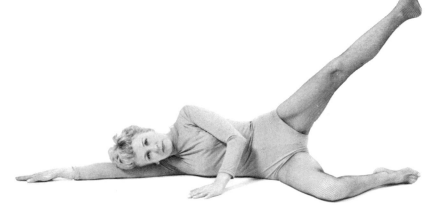

2. Raise the top leg toward the ceiling, with toes pointing up.

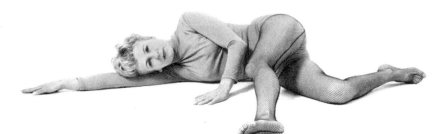

3. Now swing the leg forward to the floor and toward chest.

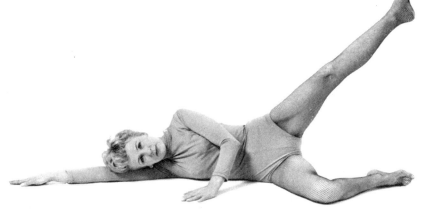

4. Raise the leg up toward ceiling again.

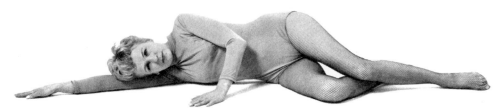

5. Lower leg back down to floor, with knee slightly bent.

Do exercise 10 times. Then roll over onto your other side and do exercise 10 times more.

53

"Five for Good Measure"

UPPER HIPS

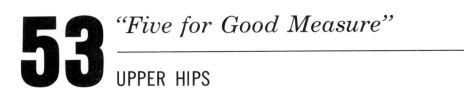

1. Lie on your side, with head resting on underneath outstretched arm. Place hand of other arm on the floor in front of chest for support. Keep your legs straight. Point toes.

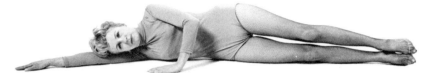

2. Keep legs together and raise them up off the floor about 2″. Hold.

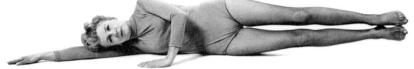

3. Raise 2″ more. Hold.

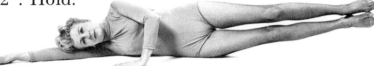

4. Lower both legs about 2″. Hold.

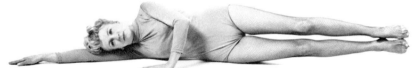

5. Lower legs to floor. Relax.

Do exercise 5 times. Roll over to other side and do 5 times more. Gradually try to increase exercise to 10 times.

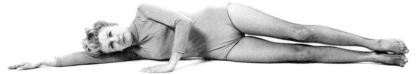

54 *"Five for Good Measure"*

UPPER HIPS

1. Stand with feet apart and knees bent slightly. Hips "tucked" under. Arms over your head. Clasp hands and turn palms up.

2. You are going to circle your body with your arms. Start by doing a deep-knee bend and bringing the clasped hands down in front of right foot. Continue the motion and bring the hands between your feet. Then swing arms to left foot. Now circle the arms to the left of body and on up over your head. (Keep knees bent as you circle down and around.)

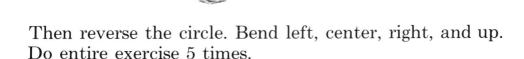

Then reverse the circle. Bend left, center, right, and up. Do entire exercise 5 times.

55 *"Five for Good Measure"*

UPPER HIPS

1. Sit on the floor, legs straight and apart, knees bent slightly. Raise your arms above your head. Clasp hands and turn palms up.

2. Twist your body to the right. Bend and bring right elbow down to right knee.

3. Come back up to a sitting position, with arms above head.

4. Twist to the left, bend and bring left elbow down to left knee. Come back up, with arms above head.

Don't force the bend—be loose and relaxed.

Do exercise 12 times.

56 *"Five for Good Measure"*

BUTTOCKS AND THIGHS

The buttocks and thighs are the most difficult part of the body to reduce, but it can be done.

Buttocks and Front and Back of Thighs

To hasten the reduction as you firm the buttocks and the front and back of thighs, you will need to do three things: (1) Increase (beyond Maintenance level) the number of times you do Exercises 25 and 26. (2) Add ankle weights to your legs as you do the Maintenance level of Exercise 15. (3) Add all of the exercises in this Buttocks and Thighs unit to your daily program, using ankle weights on your legs while doing Exercise 57.

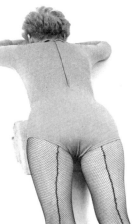

1. Lie face-down on the floor, with a pillow under your stomach, and head resting on hands.

2. Draw the buttocks together as tightly as possible. Hold. Then release the muscles gradually. Don't let go all at once. It's let go a little; hold; release a little more; hold; release a little more. Do exercise 10 times.

NOTE: Never lie face-down without a pillow under your stomach; this is the only way you can be sure of not straining back muscles.

---

57 *"Five for Good Measure"*

BUTTOCKS AND THIGHS

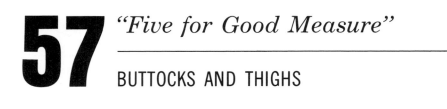

1. Lie on your side, with head resting on outstretched underneath arm. Place hand of other arm on the floor in front of your chest, for support. Bend underneath leg. Top leg is straight.

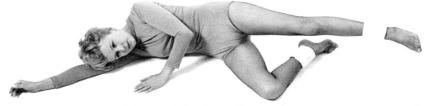

2. Raise the top leg hip level.

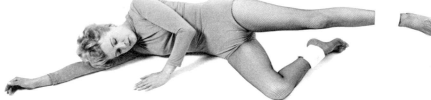

3. Now bend the leg and bring the knee to your chest.

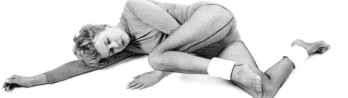

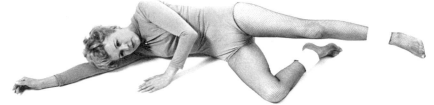

4. Straighten leg back to hip level.

Bend and straighten top leg 15 times without bringing it back to floor. Then roll over and do exercise 15 times on other side.

58 *"Five for Good Measure"*

BUTTOCKS AND THIGHS

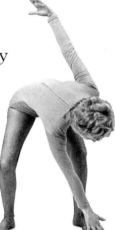

1. Stand with legs wide apart. Bend knees slightly and "tuck" hips under. Arms out shoulder level. Palms up.

2. Touch right hand to left foot, bending knees more as you do so, and extend left arm out back.

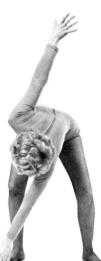

3. Come back up, with arms out and palms up. *Waist back. Ribs up. Ears up.*

4. Now touch left hand to right foot, bending knees more as you do so, and extend right arm out back.

5. Come back up again, as in position 3.

Do exercise 16 times.

59 *"Five for Good Measure"*

BUTTOCKS AND THIGHS

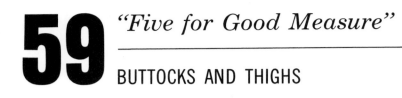

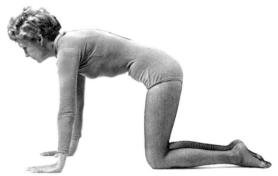

1. Get down on your hands and knees.

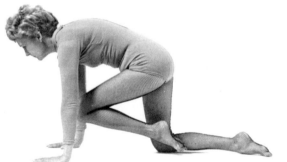

2. Bend your left knee toward chest.

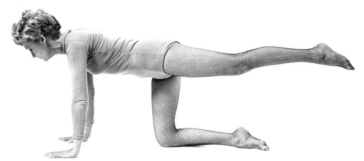

3. Extend leg out back—no higher than your buttock.

Do this with left leg (to chest and then extended back, without touching knee to floor) 10 times. Change legs and also do 10 times. Gradually try to increase to 20 times for each leg.

60 *"Five for Good Measure"*

BUTTOCKS AND THIGHS

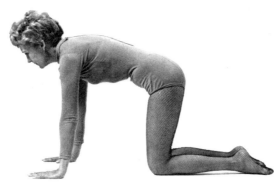

1. Get down on your hands and knees.

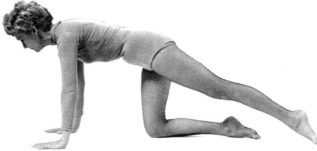

2. Extend one leg out back, with the foot resting on the floor.

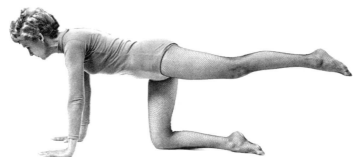

3. Raise straight leg up to hip level—not above.

4. Lower leg to floor. Do 10 times.

Change legs and also do 10 times. Gradually try to increase exercise to 20 times for each leg.

61 *"Five for Good Measure"*

OUTSIDE OF THIGHS

To hasten the reduction as you firm the outside of thighs, you will need to do three things: (1) Increase (beyond Maintenance level) the number of times you do Exercise 23. (2) Add ankle weights to your legs as you do the Maintenance level of Exercise 6. (3) Add all of the exercises in this unit to your daily program, using ankle weights on your legs while doing Exercises 62, 63 and 65.

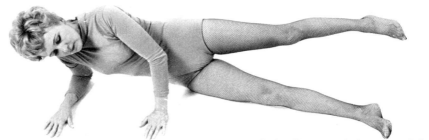

1. Lie on your side, in slight semicircle position, with the upper part of body raised and supported on elbow of underneath arm and hand of top arm. With legs apart and kept straight, raise them so that underneath leg is about 2″ from floor.

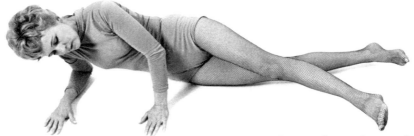

2. Keeping the legs raised, alternately swing them back and forward as if you were walking stiff-legged. Don't swing legs back beyond hip.

Do 25 times. Then roll over and do exercise 25 times on other side.

62 *"Five for Good Measure"*

OUTSIDE OF THIGHS

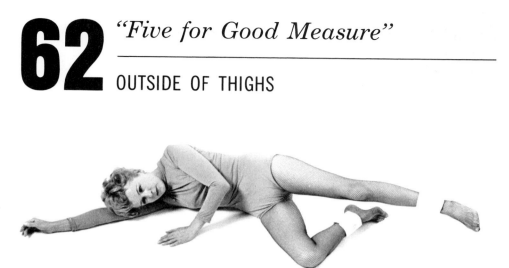

1. Lie on your side, with head resting on outstretched underneath arm. Place hand of other arm on the floor in front of chest, for support. Bend your underneath leg, but keep the top leg straight.

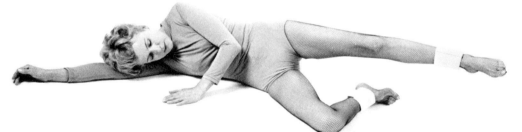

2. Now raise your top leg so it is level with your hip.

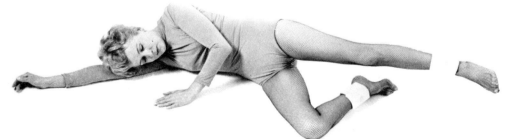

3. Bring leg forward 4″; then move it back 4″.

Do 15 times. Then roll over and do exercise 15 times on other side.

63 *"Five for Good Measure"*

OUTSIDE OF THIGHS

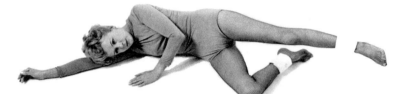

1. Lie on your side, with head resting on outstretched underneath arm. Place hand of other arm on the floor in front of chest, for support. Bend your underneath leg, but keep the top leg straight.

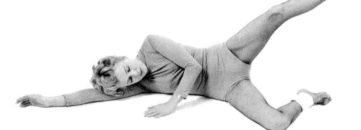

2. Raise top leg—with toes pointing up—as far as you can.

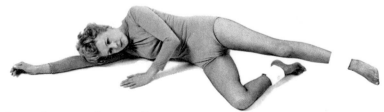

3. Then lower it to floor.

Do exercise 15 times. Then roll over and do exercise 15 times on other side.

64

"Five for Good Measure"

OUTSIDE OF THIGHS

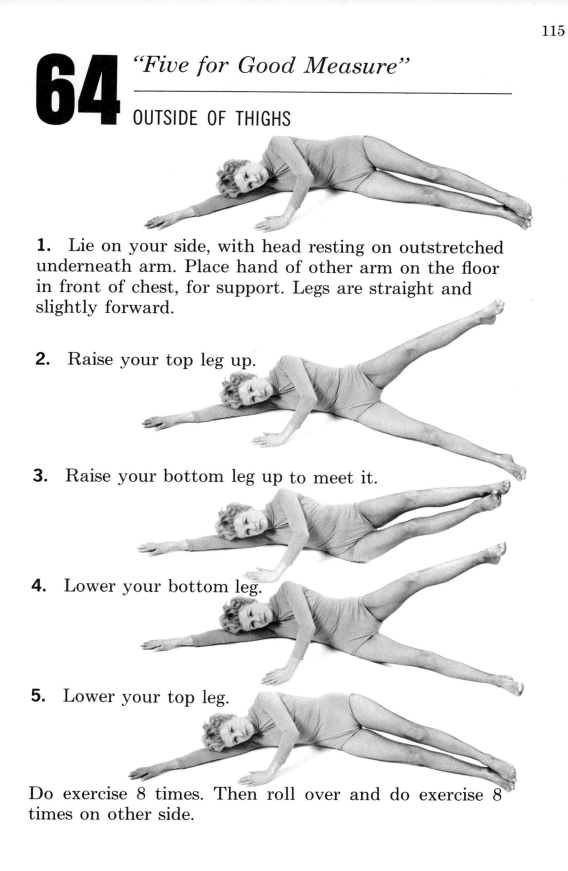

1. Lie on your side, with head resting on outstretched underneath arm. Place hand of other arm on the floor in front of chest, for support. Legs are straight and slightly forward.

2. Raise your top leg up.

3. Raise your bottom leg up to meet it.

4. Lower your bottom leg.

5. Lower your top leg.

Do exercise 8 times. Then roll over and do exercise 8 times on other side.

65 *"Five for Good Measure"*

OUTSIDE OF THIGHS

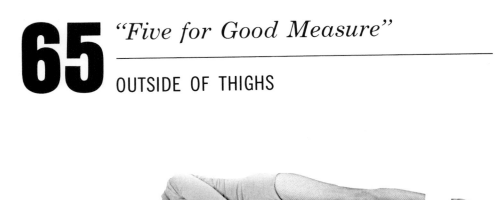

1. Lie on your side, with head resting on outstretched underneath arm. Place hand of other arm on the floor in front of chest, for support. Bend your underneath leg.

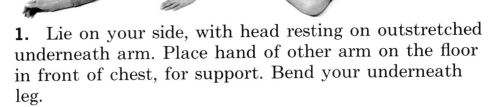

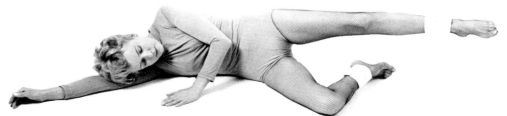

2. Now raise your top leg level with your hip. Hold.

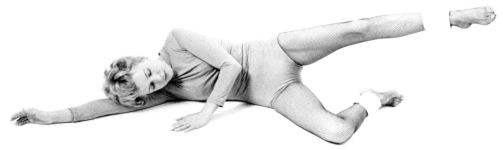

3. Raise your top leg up 2″ more. Hold.

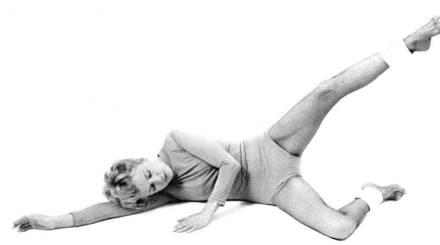

4. Now raise it up 2″ more. Hold.

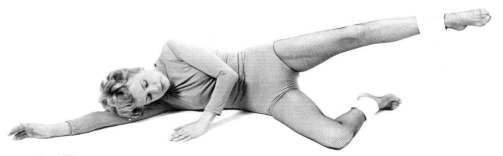

5. Then lower the leg 2″. Hold.

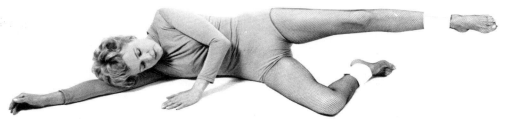

6. Lower 2″ more. Hold. At this point, the leg should again be level with your hip, ready to begin going up again.

Do exercise 8 times. Then roll over and do exercise 8 times on other side.

66

"Five for Good Measure"

INSIDE OF THIGHS

To hasten the reduction as you firm the inside of thighs, you will need to do two things: (1) Add ankle weights to your legs as you do the Maintenance level of Exercises 16, 17 (Parts I and II) and 18. (2) Add all of the exercises in this unit to your daily program, using ankle weights on your legs while doing Exercises 68 and 70.

1. "Stand" on your knees, feet together, knees apart, hips "tucked" under, arms relaxed at sides.

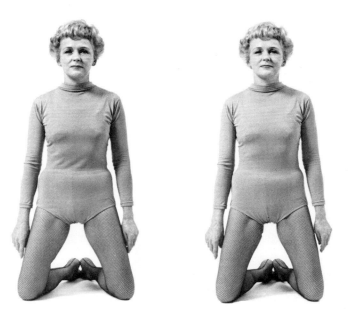

2. Now press your knees into the floor and try to bring them together. The knees will not come together but you will feel the inside of the thighs pull up and tighten. Hold for 5 counts. Relax and repeat 10 times.

67 *"Five for Good Measure"*

INSIDE OF THIGHS

Sit on the floor. Bend the knees and bring soles of feet together. Place arms slightly behind you and support your weight on your hands.

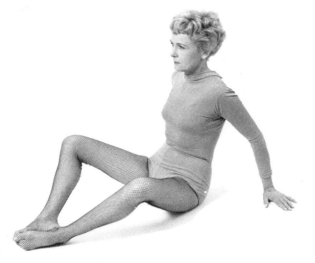

Roll pelvis backward. Pull stomach in tight. Press the soles of feet together. Press knees down, and keep pressing them toward the floor. Relax, then repeat as often as you like.

68

"Five for Good Measure"

INSIDE OF THIGHS

1. Lie on your back, with arms extended on floor, shoulder level. Palms up. Legs straight.

2. Now raise the right leg slightly off the floor and turn knee out.

3. Swing leg out to the right as far as you can.

4. Swing leg back, keeping it slightly off the floor.

Without lowering leg to floor, do exercise 10 times. Then do exercise 10 times with other leg.

69 *"Five for Good Measure"*

INSIDE OF THIGHS

For this exercise you will need a sponge rubber ball (see page 7).

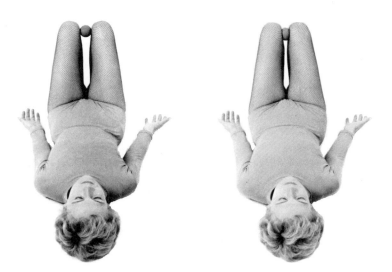

1. Lie on your back with knees bent. Keep feet together on floor and close to hips. Place the ball between your knees and . . .

2. Squeeze the ball by pressing the knees together. Hold. Relax.

Do exercise 20 times.

70 *"Five for Good Measure"*

INSIDE OF THIGHS

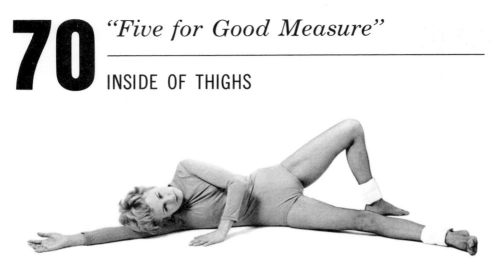

1. Lie on your side, with head resting on outstretched underneath arm. Place hand of other arm on the floor in front of chest, for support. Bend your top leg, placing foot firmly on the floor, knee pointing up toward ceiling. Bring your other leg out at a slight angle and keep it straight.

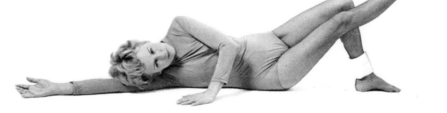

2. Slowly raise straight leg up to the bent knee.

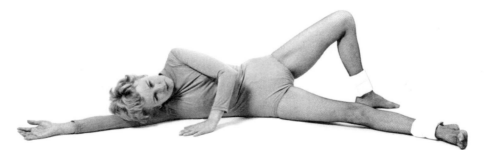

3. Lower straight leg to the floor. Repeat exercise 8 times. Then roll over and do exercise 8 times on other side.

71 "Five for Good Measure"

EXTRA BEAUTIFICATION

If your body is well proportioned, but you think your posture, ankles, knees or legs are less than perfect, you will find exercises here to help alleviate these imperfections which may be making you self-conscious.

FOR IMPROVING POSTURE / PART I

1. Stand against the wall—heels 4" out from wall, feet 4" apart and parallel, toes pointing straight ahead. Arms at your sides and pressed against the wall, palms out. Knees are bent and spine is against the wall. Now separate knees further without moving feet. Hold. Push *waist back* against wall. Raise *rib cage up* away from hips. Pull *ears up,* away from shoulders. Push *shoulders back and down*. Hold.

Relax entire body. Do exercise 5 times.

2. Then slowly slide your back up the wall only as far as you can while keeping your spine at the waistline against the wall. In this position repeat above exercise 5 times.

"Five for Good Measure"
EXTRA BEAUTIFICATION

FOR IMPROVING POSTURE / PART II

1. With a book on top of your head, stand against the wall—heels 4″ out from wall, feet 4″ apart and parallel, toes pointing straight ahead. Arms at your sides and pressed against the wall, palms out.

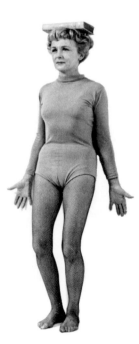

Bend knees slightly. Separate knees further without moving feet. Push *waist back* against wall. "Tuck" hips under. Raise *rib cage up* away from hips. Pull *ears up* away from shoulders. Push *shoulders back and down*.

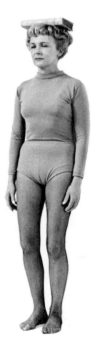

2. Now let arms hang loose at your sides. Lean slightly forward, pulling head and upper back away from wall.

3. Walk away from wall. Keep knees relaxed, hips "tucked" under. Lean slightly forward, feet pointing straight ahead. Keep arms relaxed and loose. Maintaining this position, walk across the room.

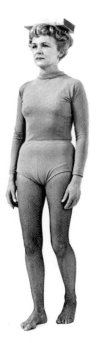

Remember—as you walk:
Knees relaxed, slightly bent.
Hips "tucked" under.
Lean slightly forward.
Rib cage up, away from hips.
Ears up, away from shoulders.
Shoulders back and down. (As you pull down, they come slightly forward.)
Arms are slightly forward.

Do exercise 5 times.

72 *"Five for Good Measure"*

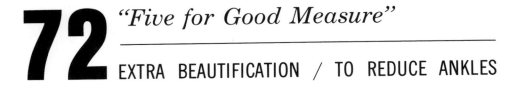

EXTRA BEAUTIFICATION / TO REDUCE ANKLES

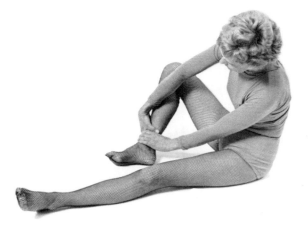

Sit on the floor, knees bent and turned out. Pull
right leg up, bring right foot up near knee of left leg.
Grab ankle of right leg with both hands. Twisting back
and forth in a wringing movement, massage the ankle
area from the bone up to the calf, lifting the hands
between each wringing movement. Repeat, starting
at the ankle bone. Don't massage down—always up.
Do 8 times. Change legs and massage ankle of the
other leg same number of times.

73 *"Five for Good Measure"*

EXTRA BEAUTIFICATION / TO REDUCE ANKLES

1. Lie down on the floor, with Turkish towels (see Exercise 15) under hips. Arms extended at shoulder level. Palms up. Bend knees over chest.

2. Straighten one leg up toward ceiling. Bring this leg toward floor, then start other leg toward ceiling as you bend and bring first leg back over chest. These movements simulate the peddling of a bicycle. As the legs move, flex the foot of the raised leg and point the toe of the bent leg.

Do exercise until ankles get tired.

Keep your legs up over your chest; don't let them drop all the way to the floor.

74 *"Five for Good Measure"*

EXTRA BEAUTIFICATION / TO REDUCE ANKLES

1. Sit on the floor, arms extended behind back, hands on floor for support. Bend knees and bring feet close to hips.

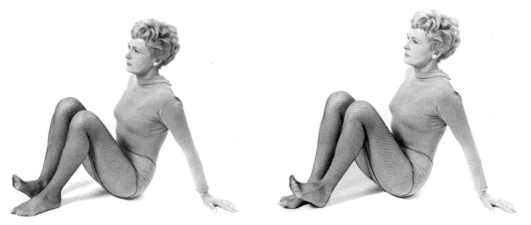

2. Then flex ankles, one at a time, first right, then left. Keep heels on floor. Do until ankles are tired.

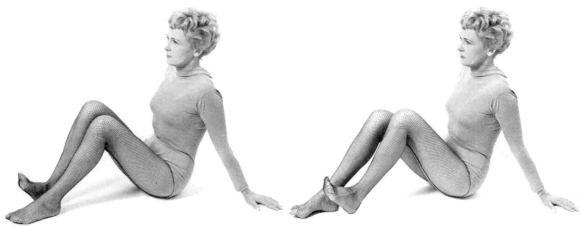

3. Slide feet down about 4″ and repeat exercise.

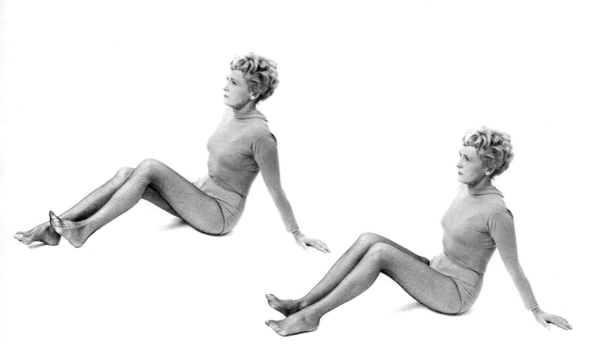

4. Slide feet down about 4″ more and repeat exercise.

5. Then, with legs almost straight, repeat exercise again.

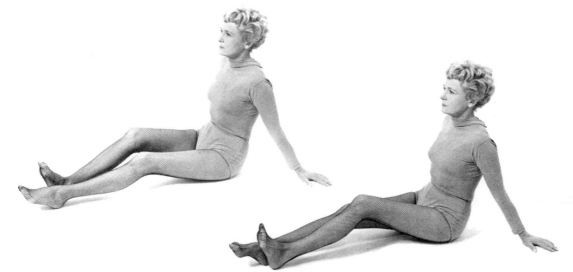

Bring legs back, feet close to hips, and repeat entire sequence 5 times. Keep the feet loose and relaxed throughout the exercise.

75 *"Five for Good Measure"*

EXTRA BEAUTIFICATION / TO REDUCE ANKLES

Lie on the floor, with Turkish towels (see Exercise 15) under hips. Arms out shoulder level. Palms up.
Raise legs up in the air and apart, feet over chest, knees relaxed.

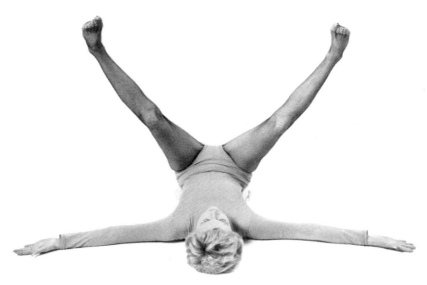

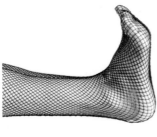

Flex feet . . .

Then point toes.

Keep this movement fast and loose.

Do until ankles are tired.

76 *"Five for Good Measure"*

EXTRA BEAUTIFICATION / TO REDUCE KNEES

1. Lie on the floor on your back, arms extended at shoulder level. Palms up. Knees bent. Feet on floor close to hips.

2. Now raise the right leg. Keep it bent and turn the knee out.

3. Then straighten and bend the leg.

Do exercise 15 times. Then change legs and do exercise with the other leg 15 times.

77 *"Five for Good Measure"*

EXTRA BEAUTIFICATION / TO CORRECT KNOCK-KNEES AND BOWLEGS

Unless the bones are deformed, knock-knees and bowlegs are due to bad posture—that is, with reference to the legs, the constant inward rotation of the thighs causes the knees to turn in and the calves of the legs to turn out. In correct posture, the hips are "tucked" under, which causes a slight outward rotation of the thigh.

PART I

1. Sit on floor, with arms extended behind your back and hands on the floor, for support. Bend the knees and bring the soles of your feet together.

2. Keeping the soles together, push the knees down toward the floor. Slowly slide feet down away from your body as far as you can, keeping the feet together, knees pressing down toward floor.

Then, one at a time, bring legs back to starting position. Do exercise 10 times.

PART II

Sit on the floor, with arms extended behind your back and hands on the floor, for support. Legs straight and together. Feet together.

Now, bend knees up slightly. Try to turn the knees out and bring the calves together, keeping heels on floor and insides of feet as close together as possible. Hold. Relax. Do exercise 10 times.

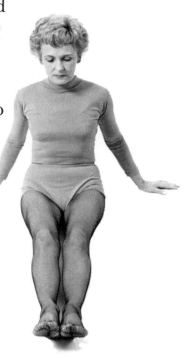

PART III

Stand with feet close together and firmly planted on the floor; knees slightly bent. "Tuck" hips under. Turn the knees out and pull the calves of legs together. Knees should barely touch. Hold. Relax. Do exercise 10 times.

This can be done any time you think of it; while waiting for a bus, elevator, etc.

SECTION III

IMPROVING WHILE MOVING—
ALL DAY, EVERY DAY

Doing exercises every day will help your muscles gain strength and tonus, so that they will begin to operate in tune with one another and thus bring "gracefulness" to the total body. But to have absolute gracefulness— that is, total coordination—you may need to break some lifelong standing, walking, sitting and movement habits.

Bad posture and bad body-movement habits are at the root of many figure faults and are, also, the cause of aches and pains—especially those in the small of the back and at the back of the neck. So in addition to your exercising, correct posture and movements ALL DAY, EVERY DAY—as you sit at a desk, do household chores, watch television, walk and stand—will help you to gain, more easily and quickly, your perfectly pro- portioned and healthy body which moves with grace.

Through the lessons in this section you will become aware of bad posture and movement habits, and learn how to correct them and replace them with new good habits. It is as important for you to act upon the sug- gestions in this section as it is for you to continue to do your exercises daily. You will be exercising only 30 minutes a day. You will be sitting, standing, moving throughout the day. Moving correctly is just as easy as moving incorrectly, once you change your habits. With correct movements "all day, every day" you can bring yourself closer to a better shape in "every way."

78 *"Improving While Moving"*

AN OUNCE OF CURE FOR ACHING BACKS

Those who have bad backs, and those who want to avoid getting one, need to be aware of the movements they make all day, every day. Tired backs, back strain and aching backs are most often generated by bad posture and incorrect body movements. People who arch their backs while donning clothes, sitting, reaching, standing, lifting or rising from a prone position are literally asking for back trouble.

Improving While Lifting

Never keep your knees hyperextended (stiff) when you touch your fingers to the floor to do an exercise or lift an object. When knees are tightly locked, the entire lifting job must be taken over by the muscles in the lower back. Just bringing your body to an upright position will be a strain to lower back muscles, and adding the weight of an object to the chore might be the proverbial straw that "breaks" your (rather than the camel's) back. The lower back muscles need help when lifting. You can get this help by bending your knees as you "toe-touch" or pick up objects. Bent knees force the leg and thigh muscles to share the "lifting" work.

WRONG

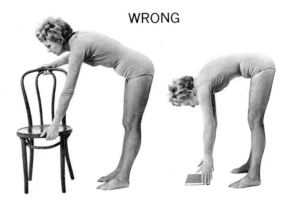

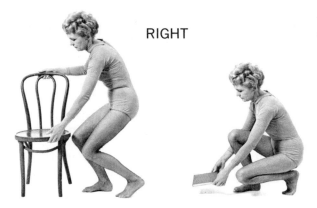

RIGHT

In addition to preventing possible strain on lower back muscles, picking up objects from the floor with bended knees helps to contour the muscles of the hips and thighs, and the same will be true when you are:

Reaching

WRONG   RIGHT

Pushing and Pulling

WRONG   RIGHT

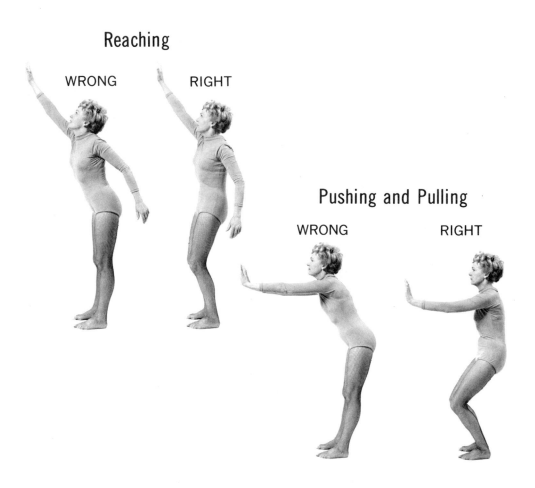

Improving While Rising from a Prone Position

Never rise from a prone position by simultaneously lifting both legs up in the air and then whisking them downward to bring yourself to a sitting position. This will force your back to arch, which puts a strain on the ligaments and muscles of the small of the back and distends the abdominal muscles. Raising and lowering straightened legs simultaneously while lying on your back is a gymnastic favorite. I would advise you not to do it. This action is apt to do your body more harm than it could ever do it good.

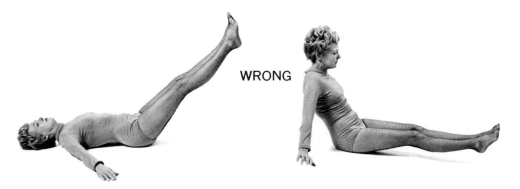

WRONG

When rising from a prone position, you should first lift your head, neck and shoulders in one smooth movement, using both elbows for support. As you come up, shift your weight to one elbow, using it for support to bring you up to a sitting position.

RIGHT

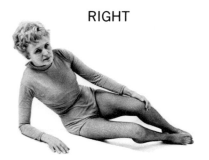

Improving While Rising from a Sitting Position

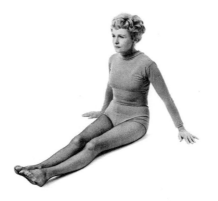

If you are sitting in bed, swing both legs over the edge so that your feet rest flat on the floor. Then proceed as you would if rising from a chair.

Improving While Rising from a Chair

To rise from a chair, put one foot a few inches in back of the other. Lean slightly forward from the waist. Push up only with the back foot, using the front foot for balance. As you rise, keep your spine straight and hips "tucked" under.

RIGHT

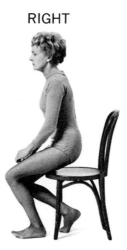

79 *"Improving While Moving"*

AN OUNCE OF CURE FOR THIGH AND BUTTOCK MUSCLES

If you are seating yourself incorrectly a hundred times a day, you are missing a great opportunity to tighten and firm thigh and buttock muscles.

Improving While Seating Yourself

If you reach out for a chair with your hips, not only does seating yourself this way look terrible, but you are not helping your body contour one bit . . . as a matter of fact, you are widening your hips.

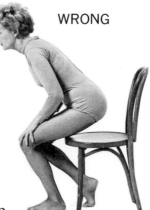

WRONG

Each time you seat yourself correctly, you will be helping to firm and tighten the muscles of the thighs and buttocks. To seat yourself correctly, stand close to a chair (bed, sofa). Place one foot behind the other. Now "tuck" your hips under, lean slightly forward from the waist and lower yourself gently into the chair.

RIGHT

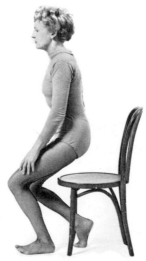

If you want proof of which seating movement best works your thigh muscles: hold your hands on your thighs as you seat yourself the right way, and the wrong way.

Improving While Sitting

WRONG   RIGHT

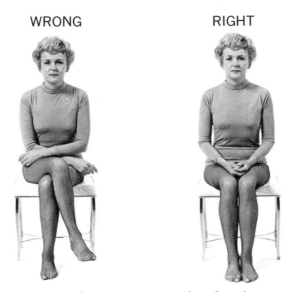

Don't cross your legs as you sit, for it cuts off circulation to the lower leg, which can cause swelling around ankles and knees.

Always sit squarely on both hips, *waist back, ribs up,* neck stretched up from the shoulders, with *shoulders* pulled *back and down,* chin at right angle to neck. Holding your torso in this position will firm and tighten the muscles of the abdomen, chest, back and neck. Sitting correctly will help you to alleviate a "bay window," rounded back, "dowager's hump" and double chin.

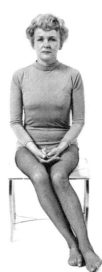

Incidentally, when posing for a picture in a seated position, move the knees to one side and your feet to the other. Place the outside foot slightly forward. This seated position will give the illusion that your hips and thighs are slimmer.

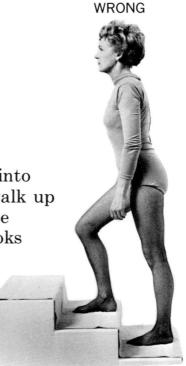

WRONG

Improving While Walking
Up and Down Stairs

You should never snap your knee into a hyperextended position as you walk up and down stairs. Snapping the knee causes the body to jerk—which looks terrible—and because the knee is stiffened, your thighs bulge, your hips stick out back and your abdomen protrudes—which isn't very pretty either.

Walking up and down stairs correctly helps to firm and trim the thighs.

RIGHT

Going Up

To walk upstairs correctly, place the whole foot on the tread of the stairs. Keep the knees slightly bent, hips "tucked" under, stomach pulled in, *ribs* pulled *up* and head held up from the shoulders. Now as you go up the stairs, feel as if you had strings attached to either side of your chest—which, like a puppet's strings, are helping to pull you up.

WRONG

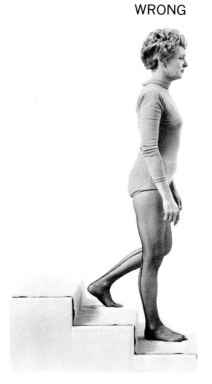

Coming Down

Your body position should be the same coming downstairs as it was going up. But as you come down, the toes should be turned slightly outward. Now feel as if you had strings attached to the top of your ears, which are helping lower you step-by-step. This will give you the sense of gliding down the stairs.

If properly done, you will have no bounce in your step as you go up and down stairs. You will therefore look better and help contour your body at the same time.

RIGHT

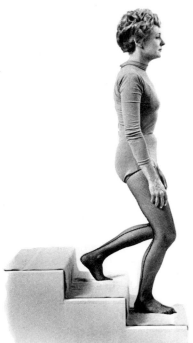

80 *"Improving While Moving"*

AN OUNCE OF CURE FOR THE WHOLE BODY

Improving While Standing

You can help tighten and firm muscles in the thighs, abdomen, buttocks, chest, back, shoulders, neck and under the chin, by standing correctly. Perfect posture will also help to correct sway-back, fallen arches, knock-knees and, unless there is a bone deformity, bowlegs. In doing the 21-Day Shape-Up Program (especially Exercises 9, 10, 11, 13, 14, 35), you have been strengthening the muscles which should help you maintain a correct standing position.

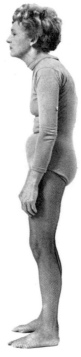

Let's take a look at what bad posture can do to your body:

If you stand with head and shoulders dropped forward, your rib cage must drop down into the abdominal region. With this stance comes a protruding abdomen (sometimes called a "bay window"), a bump at the back of the neck (known as the "dowager's hump"), sagging muscles under the chin (which gives the appearance of a double chin) and a rounded upper back. You can exercise and exercise, but to rid yourself of any one of these faults, you must also improve your posture.

WRONG

WRONG

Never stand with your knees locked into a hyperextended position. Standing stiff-kneed causes bulges to form on the outside of the thighs, the hips to stick out in the back, the back to sway, the stomach to protrude, the knees to turn in—which gives the impression of knock-knees and eventually leads to bowlegs.

When you stand, it is important to remember to keep your knees relaxed, and hips "tucked" under, for this will help to firm and trim your hips and thighs, and will aid in keeping internal organs in their proper place.

So as you stand and walk, all day, every day, remember to raise your *ribs up* away from your hips, pull your abdomen in and up under the ribs, pull your *shoulders back and down,* stretch your neck up away from your shoulders. Stand with arms relaxed and with knees slightly bent.

Always stand with your weight distributed on both feet. Constantly standing with your full weight on one leg can cause one of your hips to become higher and larger than the other.

The feet support the entire weight of the body. Tired feet and fallen arches usually indicate the body weight is being carried incorrectly. To help strengthen feet muscles you will need to do Parts I, II, III of Exercise 86, and in addition, learn how the weight of the body should be carried by the feet (see Exercise 81). Correct distribution of weight will help erase the cause of tired, aching feet as your exercises help to effect the cure.

WRONG

RIGHT

81 *"Improving While Moving"*

AN OUNCE OF CURE FOR THE FEET

Assume the correct posture position (see page 145), with knees slightly bent. Place your feet about 8″ apart, and parallel to one another, with toes pointing straight ahead. Adjust the weight of your body, forcing it equally to the heels, the outside borders and the balls of your feet. You will discover that standing with your body weight distributed in this manner will be much, much less tiring than any other way.

Improving While Walking

Your feet will tire less when walking if you keep the correct posture position (see Exercise 71) and distribute your weight evenly as you bring each foot down. Many people, when walking, tend to bring their feet out ahead of the body, making their heels carry their weight. (This is especially true of those who walk with hyperextended knees.) To walk correctly, your bended knee should be ahead of the body as you take each forward step. This action will help you to place the weight properly on your foot as it comes down. Walk with toes pointed straight ahead, and feet about 4″ apart.

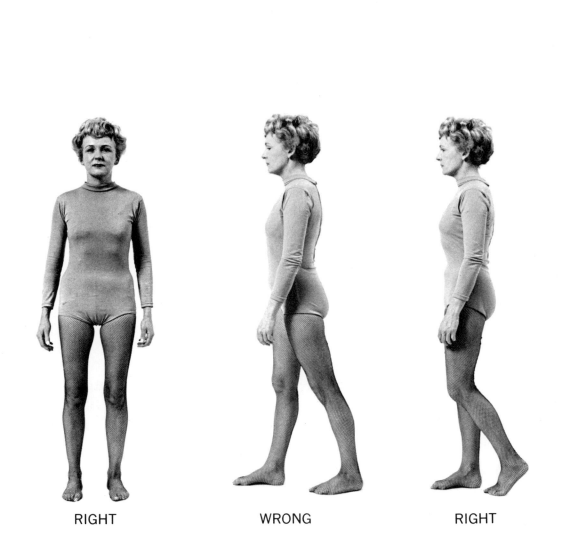

RIGHT   WRONG   RIGHT

Two-mile hikes are fine—but if you walk correctly you will also have bonus benefits: You will tone your muscles and trim your measurements. The same is true of jogging.

SECTION IV

TIRED AND NEEDY MUSCLES

During the course of a day we use some muscles more than others, and perhaps some muscles not at all. Each muscle of the body has a function to perform. When a muscle is not used, or not used enough, it will deteriorate. As muscles in various portions of the body lose vitality, they tend to make the body feel tired. Specific nerves serve each muscle and relay movement messages from the brain. When muscles are not used, or are overused, the nerves for the unused, overused or even misused muscles become tense—which results in our feeling the sensation we call nervous tension.

Continuing to do the exercise program each day will bring tone to the muscles in all parts of the body. However, an individual's activities may still require that some muscles be used more often than others, thus overtaxing them, and nervous tension may still persist. These overtaxed muscles and nerves can be relaxed—and this section will show you how. It will also give you exercises for little-used muscles in the face and hands, and show ways to get relief for tired and aching feet.

82 "Tired and Needy Muscles"

TO LOOSEN TIGHT SHOULDER MUSCLES AND RELIEVE TENSION IN THE BACK OF THE NECK

Shoulder muscles and those at the back of the neck get tired when overexercised, and tighten from nervous tension. The shoulder and neck muscles can be relaxed, and tension released, with this exercise.

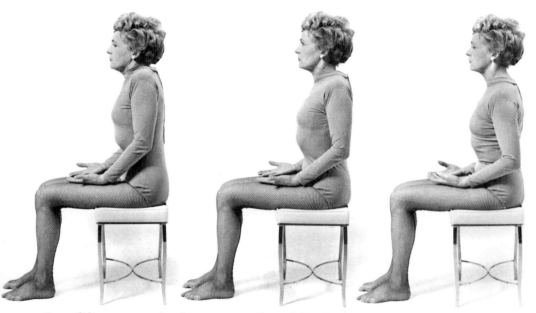

1. Sit on a chair or stool, with feet parallel and flat on the floor. Place hands on the knees. Palms up.
2. Raise shoulders up toward your ears as far as you can. In this position, pull your shoulder blades toward each other. Hold. Then relax and drop shoulders.

Do exercise at least 5 times.

NOTE: For additional exercises to loosen tight, tense shoulders and neck, see Exercises 1, 2, 10, 13, 14, 30, 31, 32.

83 *"Tired and Needy Muscles"*

TO RELIEVE BODY FATIGUE

If your whole body is feeling fatigued and you haven't time to lie down and rest, this exercise will help release body tensions and make you feel more relaxed.

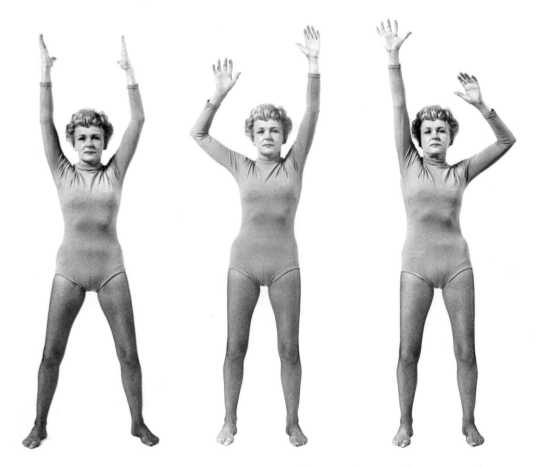

1. Stand with feet 8″ apart, with the knees bent and hips "tucked" under.

2. Raise arms over the head. Alternately stretch your arms, first one, and then the other, at least 4 times.

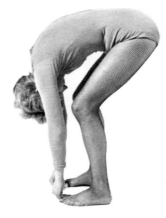

3. Let the arms drop down, and at the same time let the upper part of the body relax and drop forward. Bend your knees a little more deeply and keep the arms, neck and hands relaxed so that your head and arms are as loose as a rag doll's. In this position, sway the body back and forth several times so the loose joints move.

Do exercise at least 5 times.

NOTE: For an additional body-relaxing exercise, see Exercise 2.

84 *"Tired and Needy Muscles"*

FACE EXERCISES

The face muscles are used while talking, eating, smiling, frowning and expressing other emotional feelings. But remember, all facial expressions are not helpful; sadness and depression and tiredness cause muscles to drop. You can bring facial muscles into proper tonus, and thus ward off "aging" signs with the following exercises.

Do facial exercises in front of a mirror until you've learned the movements. Then you can do them anywhere, any time it is convenient.

PART I / UNDER-CHIN AND JOWL MUSCLES

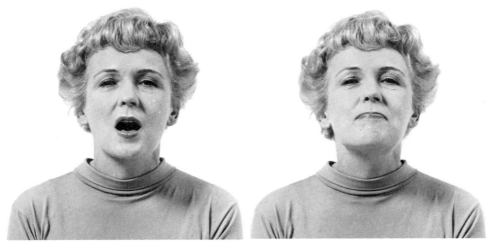

This exercise tightens the muscles, and therefore, the skin under the chin.

Say word "up," with lower lip in slight pout position. Repeat word rhythmically 20 times, or more if you like.

PART II / JOWL MUSCLES

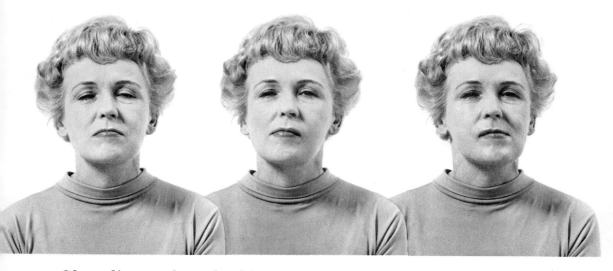

Close lips and push chin forward, then move lower jaw to right, then to left. Do not strain movement in either direction. Move side to side 20 times.

PART III / CHEEK MUSCLES

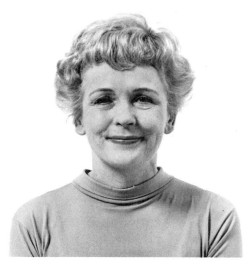

Close lips and bring them to smiling position. Keep lips in this fixed-smile position and contract the cheek muscles, pulling them up toward eyes. Repeat 20 times.

PART IV / UNDER-EYE MUSCLES

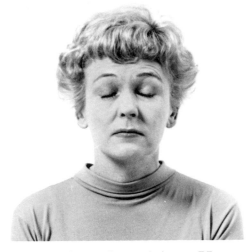

Close eyelids in a relaxed position. Keep upper lids relaxed and "pull" lower lids upward without squinting. Relax. Repeat 20 times.

PART V / UPPER-EYELID MUSCLES

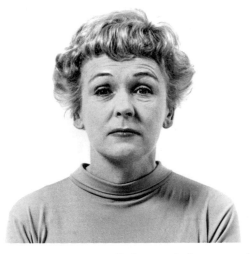

Open eyes as wide as possible, raising eyebrows as you do so, as if you'd been surprised. Hold as long as you can without strain. Then relax eyebrow muscles, but do not let upper eyelids drop. Repeat 5 times, or more if you like.

PART VI / UPPER-LIP MUSCLES

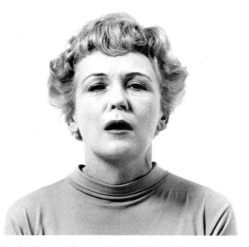

Open mouth slightly, then "pull" tip of nose down toward lips. Hold. Release. Repeat 20 times.

PART VII / UPPER-LIP MUSCLES

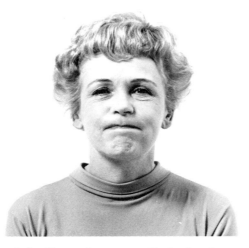

Close mouth with lips drawn slightly inward. Holding lips in this position, inflate upper lip with a puff of air. Hold. Relax. Repeat 10 times, or more if you like.

While doing any of the face exercises, try to keep muscles, other than those being exercised, relaxed.

85 *"Tired and Needy Muscles"*

HAND EXERCISES

Do hands need exercise? They do. As one grows older, the joints in the fingers tend to become stiff and knotted. One reason for this is because we use the muscles that close the hand and flex the fingers more often than we use those that extend the fingers and those that separate the fingers.

Basic position for all hand exercises: Bend elbows and hold hands up. Palms turned out.

PART I / TO LIMBER FINGERS

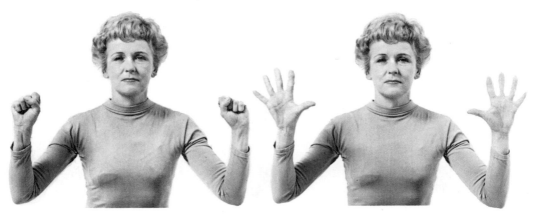

Make fists with both hands. Then open hands and extend fingers as wide as you can. Repeat 10 times.

PART II / FOR FINGER CONTROL

This exercise can be done with one hand, then the other, or with both hands at the same time.

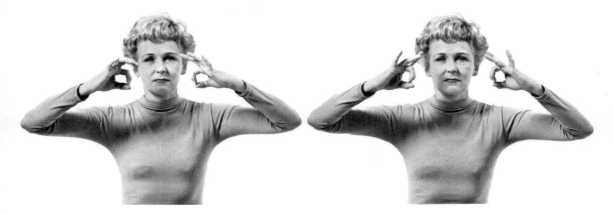

1. Make the letter "O" with the thumb and tip of first finger. Then open and extend those fingers as wide apart as possible.
2. Repeat exercise with thumb and tip of second finger.

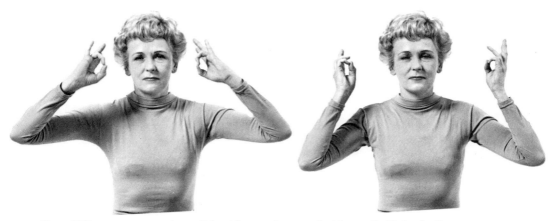

3. Then repeat with thumb and tip of third finger.
4. Then repeat with thumb and tip of fourth finger.

Do entire exercise with each hand 5 times or more.

PART III / TO STRENGTHEN FINGERS

Exercise each hand separately.

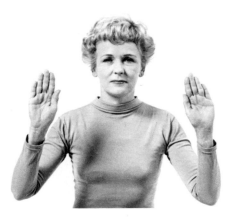

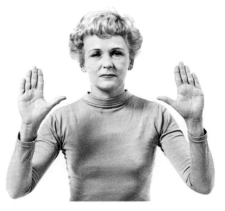

1. Straighten fingers of one hand and bring the thumb up to the fingers.

2. Separate the thumb from the first finger, still holding other fingers together.

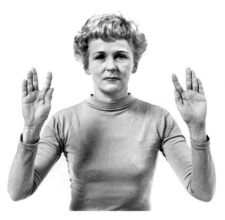

3. Bring thumb back to first finger.

4. While keeping first finger close to thumb, pull the first finger away from the second finger while holding other fingers together.

5. Bring the first finger and thumb back to starting position.

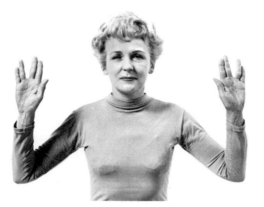

6. Now pull the third finger, keeping little finger close to it, away from the second finger without separating the thumb and first and second fingers.

7. Bring fingers back to starting position.

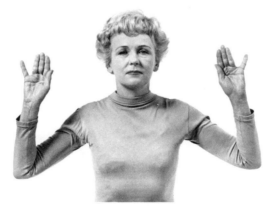

8. Keep thumb, first, second and third fingers together, and pull the little finger away from them.

9. Bring little finger back to starting position.

Repeat exercise with other hand. Do entire exercise 5 times.

86 "Tired and Needy Muscles"

FOR THE FEET

Feet ache for many reasons—ill-fitting shoes might
be the primary one, but there are other factors
which caused tired, weak feet: improper positioning
of feet as you walk, stand and sit, or the kind of
activity that requires constant standing or walking.
Whatever the reason for tired feet, exercises can
bring relief and strengthen feet muscles. As arches
fall, feet widen, which causes adults to need increas-
ingly wider or larger sizes of shoes.

Assume this basic position for all succeeding feet
exercises:

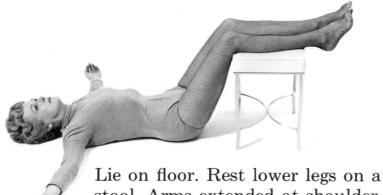

Lie on floor. Rest lower legs on a
stool. Arms extended at shoulder
level. Palms up. Keep the heels
of the feet 8″ apart and stationary.

PART I / TO STRENGTHEN THE LONGITUDINAL ARCH

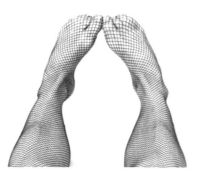 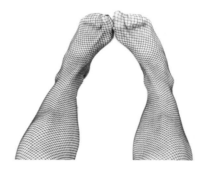

1. Turn the toes in toward each other. Hold.

2. Then pull toes up in the direction of the knees. Hold. Relax.

Do exercise 10 times.

PART II / TO STRENGTHEN METATARSAL AND LONGITUDINAL ARCHES

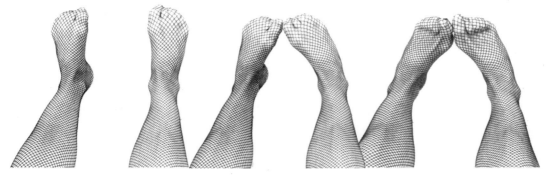

1. Grip the toes of both feet, and keep them gripped throughout exercise.

2. Bring the toes toward each other. Hold.

3. Now pull the toes up in the direction of the knees. Hold. Relax.

Do exercise 10 times.

162

PART III / TO STRENGTHEN THE METATARSAL ARCH

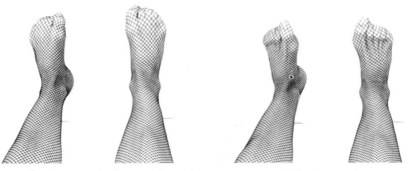

Keeping feet straight, grip the toes and bring them up in the direction of the knees. Hold. Relax.

Do exercise 10 times.

PART IV / TO STRENGTHEN MUSCLES THAT TURN FOOT IN AND OUT

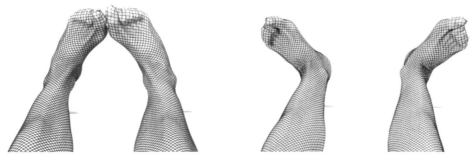

Keep feet fairly relaxed. With heels remaining stationary, move the toes of both feet toward each other, then move them away from each other. Establish a rhythmic motion of in and out.

Do exercise in and out 20 times.

NOTE: When standing, the weight of the body should be carried on the heels, the outside border and the balls of the feet. Never carry the weight of your body on the inside of your feet, for this will break down the longitudinal arches of the feet.

SECTION V
POST-PREGNANCY

During pregnancy, muscles in the abdomen, pelvic region and rib cage become stretched, and often, when physical activities are restricted, many other muscles of the body lose their tone. These special exercises are designed to strengthen the stretched—as well as the little-used—muscles and to help get the organs in the abdominal cavity back into position. They are presented here in the order I have found most beneficial for my post-pregnancy clients. However, before starting them, show them to your personal physician; check with him as to *when* you should begin and whether he feels this order is right for you.

The following program is suggested: Exercises 1–20 should be done every day for the first week; the second week, Exercises 21–23 should be added to your daily schedule. Whether following this order, or one suggested by your personal physician, work slowly and don't overdo. Remember, the muscles are weak and it will take a little time to get them back into shape. When you are able to go through all the exercises in this section with ease, again check with your personal physician, and with his permission graduate to the 21-Day Shape-Up Program—which is designed to bring the muscles in all parts of the body into tonus.

1 *"Post-Pregnancy"*

TO GET PELVIS BACK INTO POSITION

1. Assume this basic position:
Lie down on the floor on your back. Bend your knees.
Place feet together on the floor, close to hips. Keep
knees slightly apart. Place arms on floor at your sides.
Palms turned up.

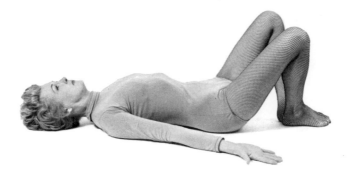

2. *Waist back.* This means: With a rolling hip movement, pull your pelvis back so the small of your back
at the waistline touches the floor.

3. Hold. *Relax.*

Do exercise 8 times.

2 *"Post-Pregnancy"*

TO STRAIGHTEN THE SPINE

1. Assume basic position (see facing page). *Waist back.*

2. *Ribs up.* This means: Pull your ribs up away from your hip bones so that you get the greatest distance possible between ribs and hip bones without lifting your spine from the floor.

3. *Ears up.* This means: Feel as if someone is holding the top of your ears and is thus stretching your neck up away from your shoulders while you are keeping your chin at a right angle to your neck.

4. *Shoulders back and down.* This means: Keep your shoulders as flat on the floor as you can, and at the same time pull them down toward your feet; feel as though your arms were being pulled by your little fingers.

5. Hold. *Relax.*

Do exercise 5 times.

NOTE: **Waist back. Ribs up. Ears up. Shoulders back and down. Relax.**

These are the key phrases which appear in many of the exercises that follow. When you read these words, they will be calling for the actions described above. Memorize these phrases and their meanings. Only by acting upon them can you bring yourself back to perfect shape.

---

3 *"Post-Pregnancy"*

TO STRENGTHEN ABDOMINAL MUSCLES

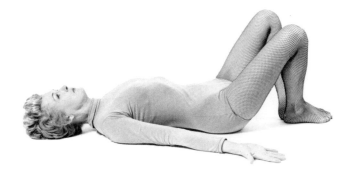

1. Assume basic position (see page 164). Now: *Waist back. Ribs up. Ears up. Shoulders back and down.*

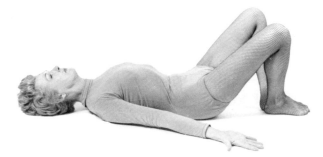

2. Blow all the air you can out of your lungs. Compress your lips and hold your breath.

3. Before inhaling again, pull stomach in, then up under ribs. Hold. Hold. Hold. *Relax.*

Do exercise 6 times.

4 *"Post-Pregnancy"*

TO LENGTHEN WAISTLINE BY LIFTING RIBS

1. Lie on the floor on your back, with arms extended over the head, and elbows relaxed. Palms turned up.

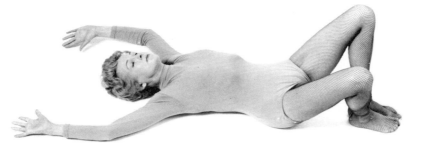

2. Bend your knees and place feet together on the floor close to hips. Keep knees separated. Now: *Waist back.*

3. Pull the stomach in. Keeping spine on floor, stretch up with left hand. Hold. Then relax. Next, stretch up with right hand. *Stretch* so you feel your rib cage move. Keep arms as close to floor as possible.

Stretch each arm 8 times.

Do the exercise with loose and relaxed movements. Do not tense. Do not push stomach out.

5 "Post-Pregnancy"

TO STRENGTHEN MUSCLES IN PELVIS AND ABDOMEN

1. Lie on your back, arms extended on floor, shoulder level. Palms up. Bend knees. Place feet on floor close to hips. Feet together. Knees slightly apart.

2. NOW: *Waist back. Ribs up. Ears up. Shoulders back and down.* Holding this position, bend your right knee up toward your chest.

3. Raise the right leg, straightening it as you do so.

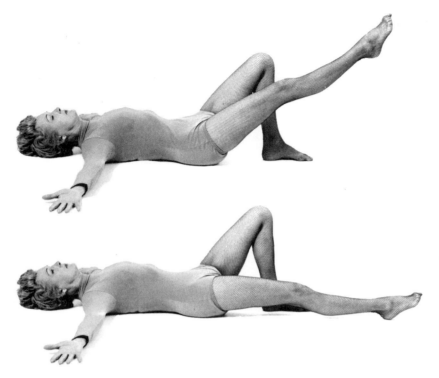

4. *Slowly* lower the leg down to the floor, *keeping spine on the floor* and *stomach pulled in tight.*

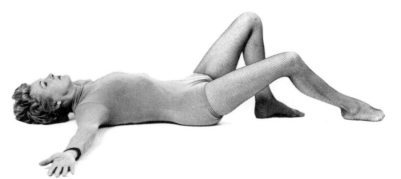

5. Then slowly bend the knee and return leg to its starting position.

Repeat same movements with left leg.

Do exercise 5 times with each leg.

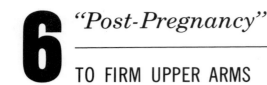

6 *"Post-Pregnancy"*

TO FIRM UPPER ARMS

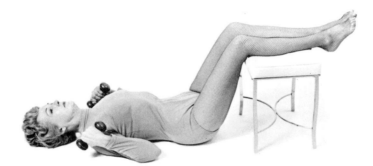

1. Lie on floor. Rest lower legs on a stool, as shown, or on a low bed, sofa or chair seat. Spine at waist should be flat on the floor. Hold a 3-pound dumbbell in each hand, with palms facing. Bend your elbows and bring arms close to your body. Keep your chin at right angle to body.

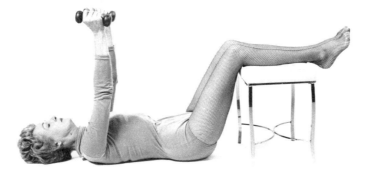

2. Straighten forearms, so hands point toward ceiling but elbows are still on floor, before slowly pushing the dumbbells up until your arms are straight. Push with a nice, smooth motion. No jerking. No snapping of elbows.

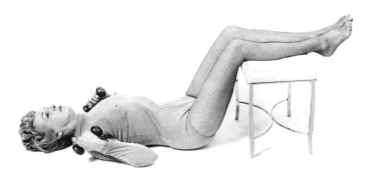

3. Slowly bring the dumbbells straight down again, bending elbows as arms move down.

Do exercise 10 times.

By keeping the fists clenched, this exercise, and the following three, can be done without dumbbells, but the arm muscles can be toned more quickly if 3-pound dumbbells are used. (See Weights, page 6.)

7 *"Post-Pregnancy"*

TO FIRM ENTIRE ARM AND BUST

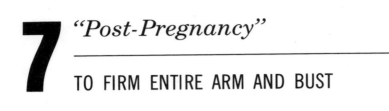

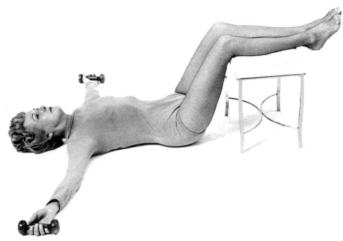

1. Lie on floor with lower legs resting on stool. *Waist back. Ears up.* Arms extended on floor, shoulder level. Backs of hands resting on floor, with a 3-pound dumbbell in each hand.

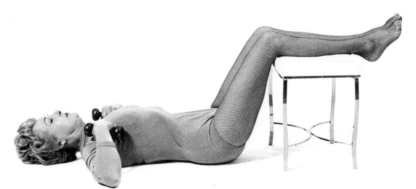

2. Bend elbows and bring dumbbells toward shoulders, keeping elbows, upper arms and shoulders on floor.

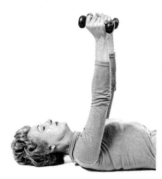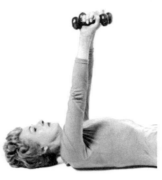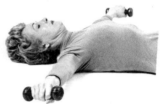

3. Straighten arms up toward ceiling, palms facing each other.

4. Turn palms out, and . . .

5. Slowly lower arms to floor.

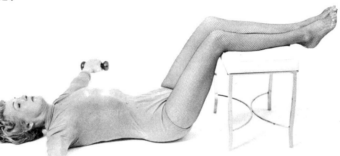

6. With dumbbells resting on floor, turn hands to . . .

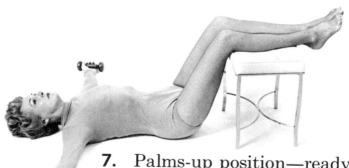

7. Palms-up position—ready to begin again.

Do exercise 10 times.

8 *"Post-Pregnancy"*

TO FIRM BUST

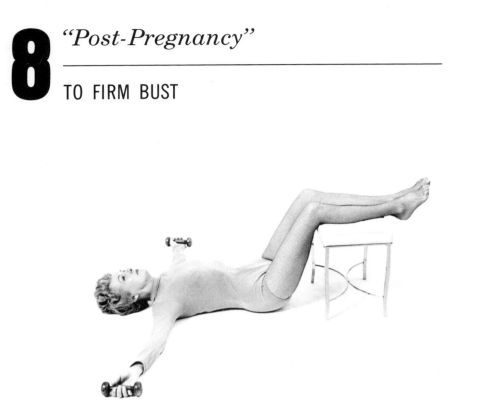

1. Lie on floor with lower legs resting on stool. *Waist back. Ears up.* Arms extended on floor, shoulder level. Backs of hands resting on floor, with a 3-pound dumbbell in each hand.

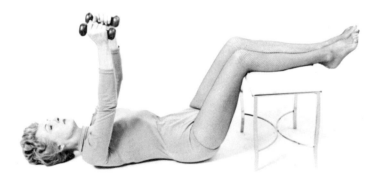

2. Keeping arms straight, slowly raise them up over chest, until . . .

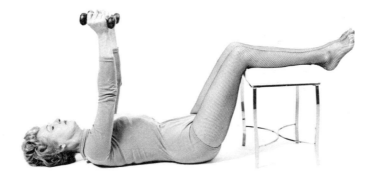

3. Dumbbells almost meet in center.

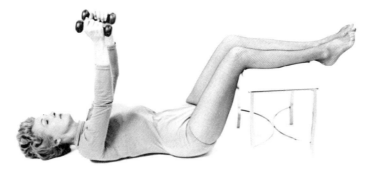

4. Still keeping arms straight, *slowly* lower them, until . . .

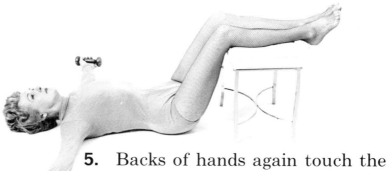

5. Backs of hands again touch the floor.

Do exercise 10 times.

9 *"Post-Pregnancy"*

TO FIRM FRONT OF UPPER ARMS

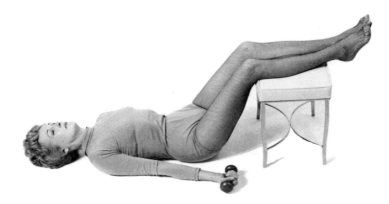

1. Lie on floor with lower legs resting on stool. *Waist back. Ears up.* Arms on floor, at your sides, close to the body. Backs of hands resting on floor, with a 3-pound dumbbell in each hand.

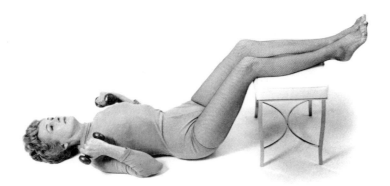

2. Slowly bend your elbows, keeping them on floor. Bring dumbbells to your shoulders.

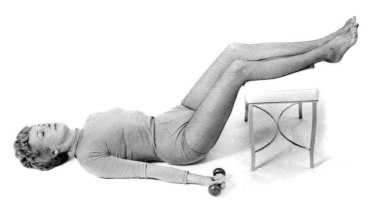

3. Slowly straighten arms and lower dumbbells back down to the floor to the starting position.

Do exercise 15 times.

10 "Post-Pregnancy"

TO FIRM ARMS AND LEGS, WAIST AND ABDOMEN

1. Lie on the floor on your back, with arms over the head, and elbows relaxed. Palms up. *Waist back*. Bend your knees and place your feet together on the floor as far from your hips as you can while comfortably holding the small of your back to the floor. Pull the stomach in.

2. Keeping your head and shoulders on floor, raise your right arm and left leg up toward ceiling. Touch right hand to left leg (DO NOT STRAIN to touch toes. Keep knees relaxed).

3. Then lower arm, keeping elbow slightly bent, to the floor. Lower leg back to its original position, with foot on floor. Push *waist back*. Pull stomach in.

4. Next, raise other arm and leg. Touch, and down. *Waist back*. Pull stomach in.

Do exercise 10 times with each leg.

11 *"Post-Pregnancy"*
TO FIRM WAIST, OUTSIDE OF THIGH AND FAT AROUND ARM SOCKET

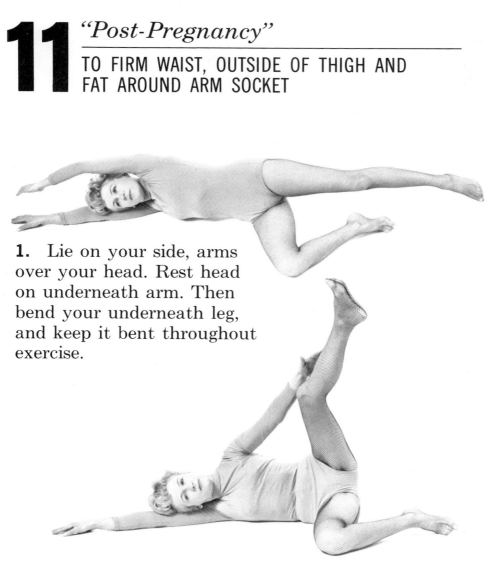

1. Lie on your side, arms over your head. Rest head on underneath arm. Then bend your underneath leg, and keep it bent throughout exercise.

2. Raise your top arm and leg toward ceiling. Touch hand to leg. (Don't try to touch toes.) Return arm and leg to original position.

3. When arm and leg return to original position, stretch top arm up behind your head. Stretch as far as you can—pull, pull, pulling your rib cage away from your hip.

Do exercise 10 times, then turn over and repeat on other side.

12 *"Post-Pregnancy"*

TO FIRM ENTIRE LEG

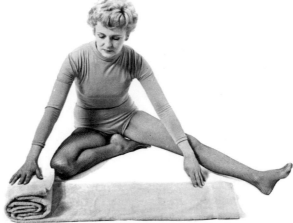

To do any exercise which requires both legs being in the air simultaneously, you must support your back. For proper back support, you will need two Turkish towels. Fold each one in half lengthwise. Roll up one folded towel. Then roll the other one around it.

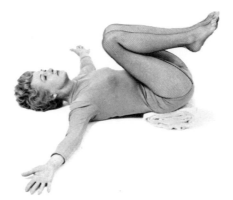

1. Lie down on floor and place rolled towels under your buttocks, adjusting roll to position that will give your back the greatest support. When towel roll is in place: Extend arms to shoulder level. Palms up. Bend both knees over your chest.

2. Straighten one leg up toward ceiling. Bring this leg toward floor, then start other leg toward ceiling as you bend and bring first leg back over chest. These movements simulate the peddling of a bicycle.

Keep your legs up over your chest; don't let them drop all the way to floor. Keep feet relaxed. Do not point toes.

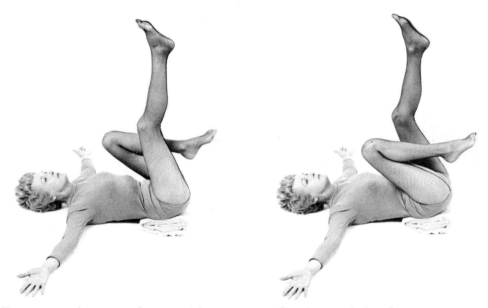

Do exercise 20 times. (Count each time right leg comes up as one complete cycle.)

NOTE: You will get more benefit from cycling on the floor than from a real bike ride. Real biking can build bulging muscles in the legs. Your simulated ride *tones* muscles and helps reduce upper-thigh bulges.

13 *"Post-Pregnancy"*

TO FIRM AND TIGHTEN FLABBY MUSCLES OF INSIDE OF THIGHS

PART I

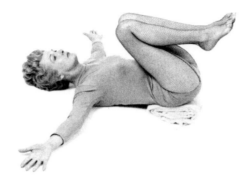

1. Lie down on floor and support your back with towels, as in previous exercise. Extend arms to shoulder level. Palms up. Bend both knees over your chest.

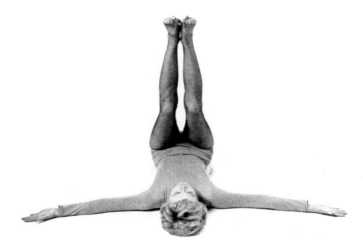

2. Now extend legs up over chest.

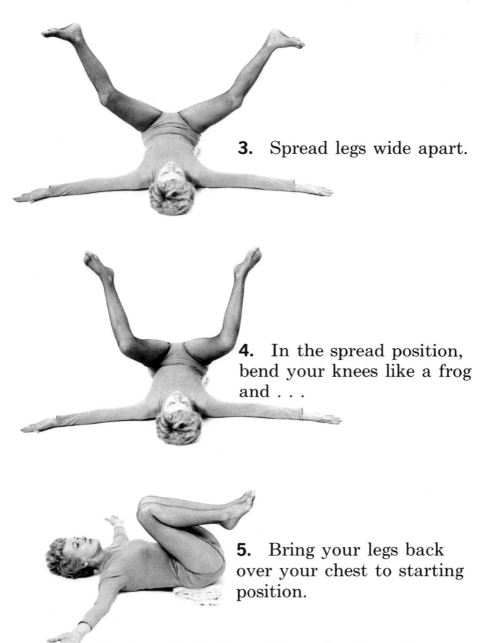

3. Spread legs wide apart.

4. In the spread position, bend your knees like a frog and . . .

5. Bring your legs back over your chest to starting position.

Do Part I 10 times. Then do Part II same number of times.

PART II / REVERSE ACTION

From starting position, reverse entire action, going from froglike position back to starting position.

14 *"Post-Pregnancy"*

TO FIRM INSIDE OF THIGHS

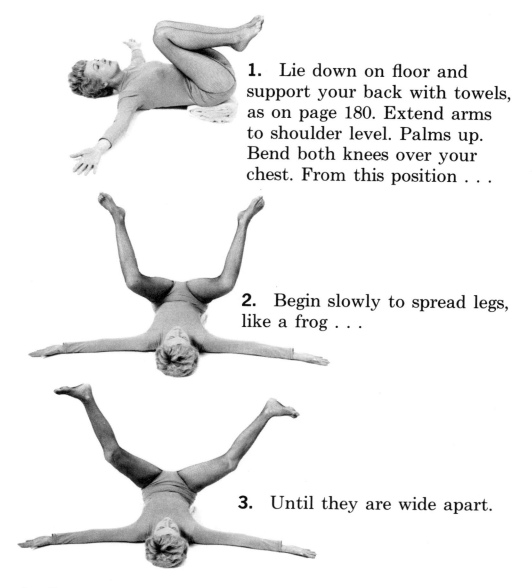

1. Lie down on floor and support your back with towels, as on page 180. Extend arms to shoulder level. Palms up. Bend both knees over your chest. From this position . . .

2. Begin slowly to spread legs, like a frog . . .

3. Until they are wide apart.

4. In one smooth movement, bend knees back to starting position.

Do exercise 10 times.

15 *"Post-Pregnancy"*

TO STRENGTHEN ABDOMEN

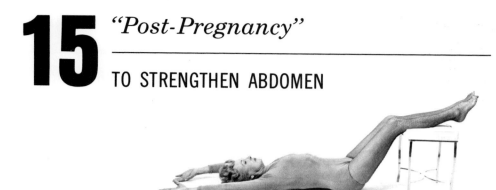

1. Lie down on the floor with lower legs resting on a stool. Arms over the head on the floor. Palms up.

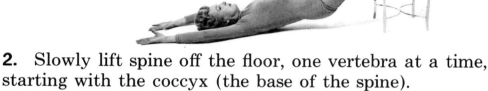

2. Slowly lift spine off the floor, one vertebra at a time, starting with the coccyx (the base of the spine).
Up, up, up.

3. When you are up, stretch from the tip of your fingers to the tip of your toes.

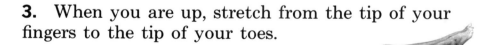

4. Then come down slowly, one vertebra at a time, starting at the top. As you come down, pull stomach in (down toward the floor). Keep hips raised until you lower small of back to floor, then bring hips down.

Do exercise 5 times.

16 *"Post-Pregnancy"*

TO FIRM UPPER BACK AND SHOULDERS

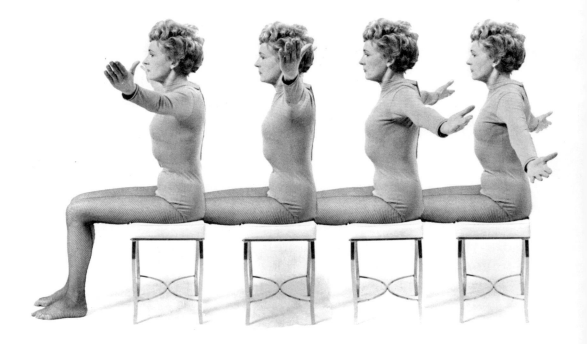

Sit on a stool with feet flat on the floor (or sit tailor-fashion on floor. See page 190). Bring arms out to shoulder level. Palms up. Now move arms in small circles, up, back and down.

Do exercise 10 times.

17 *"Post-Pregnancy"*

TO FLATTEN UPPER BACK

Sit on a stool with feet flat on the floor. Push your spine at the waistline out back. Raise both arms over your head just in front of your ears. Clasp hands and turn palms up. Keeping hands clasped in this manner, push both arms so they go behind your ears. Relax.

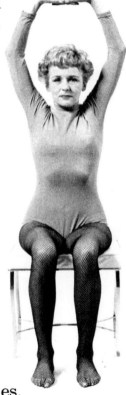

Move arms back and forth 10 times.

Don't lean back. Don't let your head come forward. Just move those arms.

18 *"Post-Pregnancy"*

TO FIRM ENTIRE LEG

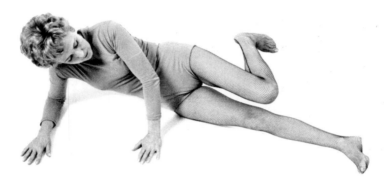

1. Lie down on your side with body in slight semicircle position, with the upper part of body raised and supported on elbow of underneath arm and hand of top arm.

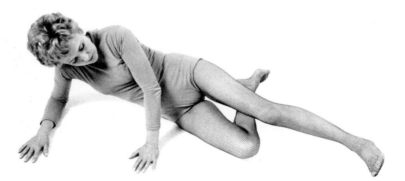

2. With both legs raised about 2″ off floor, bend and straighten legs, first one, then the other, as if you were peddling a bicycle. Pull your toes up and heels down and "pump" with your feet in this position. You will then get a pull in the calves of your legs. As you "bicycle," adjust your position on your arms so that you literally massage the side of the upper thigh with each cycling movement.

"Bicycle" 20 times. (Count each time right leg comes up as one complete cycle.) Then roll over and "bicycle" on other side for same number of times.

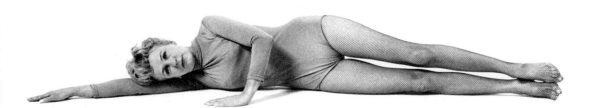

If you do not have a heavy-thigh problem, you will not need to raise the upper portion of body while cycling. Instead, lie on the floor on your side, with head resting on outstretched underneath arm. Place hand of other arm on the floor in front of chest for support. Raise legs 2″ off floor and do exercise.

19 *"Post-Pregnancy"*

TO FIRM AND TIGHTEN ARMS AND BUST

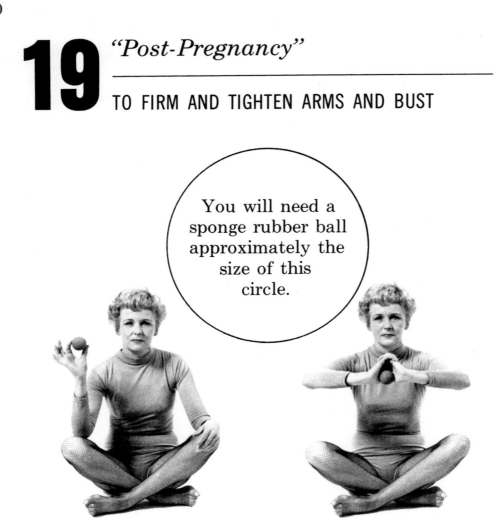

You will need a sponge rubber ball approximately the size of this circle.

PART I

Sit on a chair, or tailor-fashion on floor, as shown.

Bend your arms and bring elbows to chest height, with hands about 8" away from body. Place ball between your palms, resting it on the heels of your hands, with fingers interlocked.

Press the heels of your hands against the ball for the count of 5. Relax the pressure.

Do exercise 20 times.

PART II

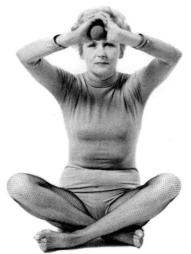

Raise hands to forehead level. Press the ball between heels of interlocked hands and hold pressure for count of 5. Then relax.

Do exercise 20 times.

PART III

Bring arms behind back, at hip level. Press the ball between heels of interlocked hands and hold pressure for count of 5. Then relax.

Do exercise 10 times.

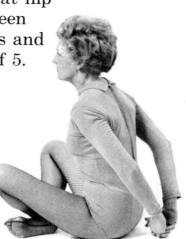

20 *"Post-Pregnancy"*

TO FLATTEN UPPER BACK AND TO FIRM BUST

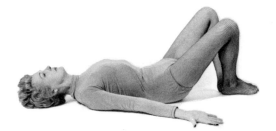

1. Lie on your back, arms at sides. Palms up. Knees bent. Feet together on floor, close to hips. Knees slightly apart. *Waist back. Ribs up. Ears up. Shoulders back and down.*

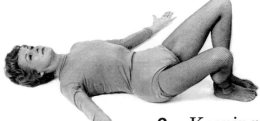

2. Keeping thumbs on floor, slowly bend your elbows and slide your arms to . . .

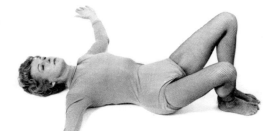

3. Shoulder level. Then stop. Check: *Waist back. Ribs up. Ears up. Shoulders back and down.*

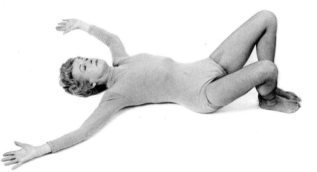

4. Keeping corrected body position, slowly slide arms on the floor . . .

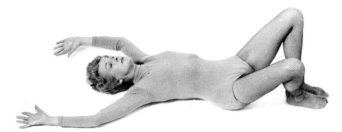

5. Up over your head, as far as you can go while keeping elbows and wrists and small of back pressed against the floor.

Now you are going to bring your arms back to the starting position in the following manner:

Keeping elbows on the floor, pull shoulders down away from ears and bring arms down 2″ (see 4). Stop. Check: *Waist back. Ribs up. Ears up. Shoulders back and down.* Then bring arms down another 2″. Stop and check body position again. Keep bringing arms down 2″ at a time until fingers reach shoulder level (see 3). Then, pulling down with your little fingers, slowly bring arms all the way down to your sides (see 1). Hold when arms are at sides and pull, pull, pull shoulders down. *Relax.*

Do exercise 5 times.

Start the following three exercises during the second week.

21 *"Post-Pregnancy"*

TO FIRM WAIST AND ABDOMEN AND TO CONTOUR UPPER HIPS

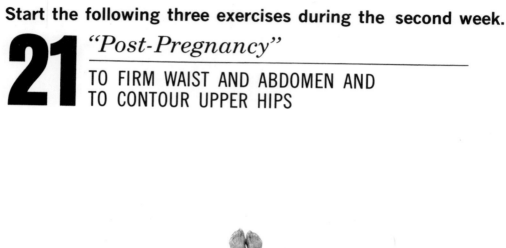

1. Lie on your back, arms extended on floor, at shoulder level. Palms up. Bend your knees up over your chest.

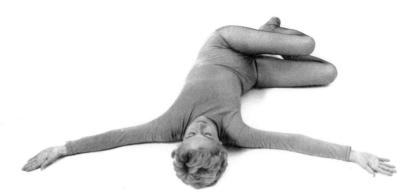

2. Keeping knees together, drop both knees to right side, all the way to the floor, and directly out from hips. Keep arms as close to floor as possible.

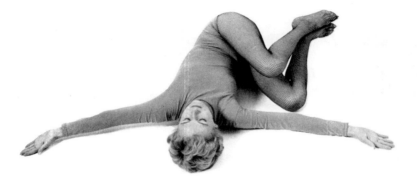

3. Keeping knees on the floor, pull them up toward elbow. Hold. From this pulled-up position:

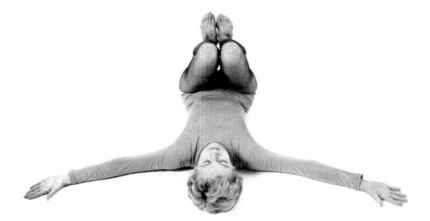

4. Roll knees back over your chest. Hold.

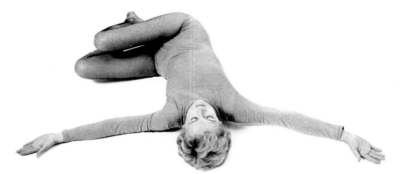

5. Drop both knees to left side directly out from hips; pull knees up toward elbow. Hold. Bring knees back over chest. Hold.

Do exercise 10 times.

22 *"Post-Pregnancy"*

TO FIRM WAIST, UPPER HIPS AND DIAPHRAGM

1. Lie on your back, arms extended on the floor at shoulder level. Palms up. Legs extended.

2. Bend your left knee and . . .

3. Cross it over your body toward the right elbow. Do this in one movement. Let the hip roll as you stretch the knee over. Keep shoulders on the floor. Bring leg back to starting position and repeat same movements with other leg.

Do exercise 8 times with each leg.

23 *"Post-Pregnancy"*
BREATHING EXERCISE FOR DIAPHRAGM AND MUSCLES BETWEEN RIBS

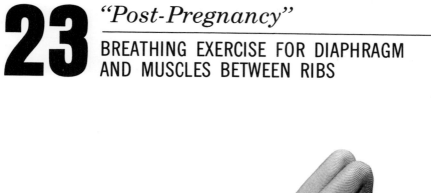

1. Lie on your back, knees bent, feet together on floor close to hips. Keep knees slightly apart. Place your hands, palms down, on your rib cage.

2. Exhale, but do not push your stomach muscles out as you do so. Instead, you should feel your rib cage moving inward. Blow all the air you can out of your lungs. Blow it out slowly.

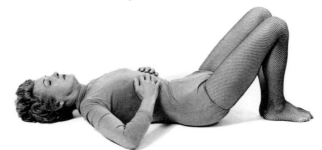

3. Inhale deeply. As the air goes into your lungs, you should feel your rib cage expand.

Throughout the exercise, your rib cage should be moving in and out, like an accordion.

Do exercise 5 times.

INDEX

All figures refer to exercise numbers except those in italic which refer to page numbers.

NOTE: Most of the exercises in this book bring many more muscles into action than those specifically mentioned. The index will guide the reader to exercises to reduce specific areas of the body—even though other muscles and areas may also be toned as a result of the natural movements.